# Praise for the First Edition

"Boris Draznin is an accomplished scientist and clinician who provides a sound scientific basis for his unique approach to the prevention and treatment of diabetes. The emphasis is placed on obesity and lifestyle modifications. Importantly, both sides of the energy balance equation—food intake and activity—are stressed. The Draznin Mile and Draznin Calorie are practical concepts that make his plan easier to follow. Dr. Draznin's numerous patient experiences exemplify his points while offering a personal and comforting encounter for the reader. An important and parting note encourages those at risk for diabetes, or with diabetes, to choose physicians with the knowledge, interest, and time to deal with this important problem."

*—Robert H. Eckel, M.D., University of Colorado Health Sciences Center*

"The prevalence of diabetes and obesity has reached epidemic proportions in America, leading to an enormous health problem. This new book by Boris Draznin will be of great help to anyone trying to deal with the problem of excess weight. It is highly readable, medically correct, and filled with useful, practical advice. Dr. Draznin carefully explains the basic concepts of calorie balance and weight control and then goes on to describe a lifestyle program that anyone can adapt to their own needs. Using his approach people will be able to take charge of their attitudes and behaviors towards calories and exercise and, thereby, take control of their weight."

*—Jerrold M. Olefsky, M.D., University of California, San Diego, School of Medicine*

"In his book, *The Thinking Person's Guide to Diabetes: The Draznin Plan*, Boris Draznin brings the same wit, excellence, and passion to the reader that he does in person. The concepts of the Draznin Calorie and the Draznin Mile bring lightness, reality, and possibility to the chore of day-to-day living with diabetes mellitus. Each reader will find his or her own path using his approach. I heartily recommend this book to all people with diabetes."

*—Gerald Bernstein, M.D., F.A.C.P., Past President, American Diabetes Association*

"*The Thinking Person's Guide to Diabetes: The Draznin Plan* is written by a world expert in diabetes and obesity, but is readily accessible by the layman. It gives practical advice to overweight individuals but is definitely not a fad diet book because it is founded on evidence-based medicine. This excellent book offers a very balanced approach to diet and exercise—it's proven to work."

*—Derek LeRoith, M.D., Ph.D., Chief of the Division of Endocrinology, Diabetes, and Bone [ . . . . . . . . . . . . . . . School of Medicine*

D0819292

# Living with Diabetes

## Dr. Draznin's Plan for Better Health

Boris Draznin, MD, PhD

OXFORD
UNIVERSITY PRESS

2008

# OXFORD
UNIVERSITY PRESS

Oxford University Press, Inc., publishes works that further
Oxford University's objective of excellence
in research, scholarship, and education.

Oxford New York
Auckland Cape Town Dar es Salaam Hong Kong Karachi
Kuala Lumpur Madrid Melbourne Mexico City Nairobi
New Delhi Shanghai Taipei Toronto

With offices in

Argentina Austria Brazil Chile Czech Republic France Greece
Guatemala Hungary Italy Japan Poland Portugal Singapore
South Korea Switzerland Thailand Turkey Ukraine Vietnam

Published by Oxford University Press, Inc.
198 Madison Avenue, New York, New York 10016

www.oup.com

Oxford is a registered trademark of Oxford University Press

Library of Congress Cataloging-in-Publication Data
Draznin, Boris.
Living with diabetes : Dr. Draznin's plan for better health / Boris Draznin.
p. cm.
Includes index.
Revised ed. of: The thinking person's guide to diabetes. 2003.
ISBN 978-0-19-534166-9
1. Non-insulin-dependent diabetes—Popular works. 2. Weight
loss—Popular works. I. Title.
RC662.18.D73 2008
616.4'62–dc22
2007052458

9 8 7 6 5 4 3 2 1

Printed in the United States of America
on acid-free paper

# Preface to the Revised Edition

Since the year 2003, when the first edition of this book was published, the epidemic of obesity has continued, unchecked by heightened public attention, hundreds of articles in scientific and popular periodicals, multitudes of broadcast news pieces about the dangers of obesity, and an unstoppable proliferation of diet books and dietary advice for children and adults. Along with obesity, the prevalence of diabetes has also continued to climb. According to one study from Canada, the number of people with diabetes in Ontario in 2005 exceeded that predicted by scientists for the year 2030. Regretfully, we are twenty-five years ahead of this sobering health prediction, and we are losing the battle with obesity and diabetes.

While we anxiously await the discovery of a magic pill that would either effectively and safely curb our appetites or prevent weight gain in some other way, I offer the Draznin Plan as a healthy and successful way to prevent and treat diabetes in most people who make a commitment to follow it.

In this revised edition of the book, I will introduce a few new steps that will make it even easier for readers to adopt the Draznin Plan and, with it, a healthier lifestyle. All of the advice given to my readers in the first edition still stands: Build an attainable and practical exercise program of three Draznin Miles per day and never buy or eat anything that contains more than 2.5 g of saturated fat or 6 g of sugar per serving.

I sincerely hope this new edition will help more people with diabetes and prediabetes join the ranks of those who have already successfully embraced the Draznin Plan and a healthier, longer life.

B. D.
Denver, Colorado
2007

# Preface to the First Edition

Not a week passes by without a story in the news media about the epidemic of obesity and type 2 diabetes in the United States. These stories appear regularly in major national news publications and on television. This epidemic is not limited to the U.S. borders; Canada, England, and other industrialized nations are experiencing these same intractable health problems.

This epidemic is real. It is frightening. It has colossal implications for the health of our population and for the healthcare system in general. Obesity and type 2 diabetes are silent killers responsible for the shortened life expectancy of many people. One of the most important complications of type 2 diabetes is the acceleration and progression of cardiovascular disease, leading to heart attack and stroke. Needless to say, these complications significantly and adversely affect both life span and quality of life.

At the same time, clinical trials have convincingly demonstrated that type 2 diabetes can be prevented. One study showed that modifications in eating habits and activity patterns effectively prevented diabetes in almost 60% of "prediabetic" patients. We have also learned that weight reduction helps control blood pressure and cholesterol problems. The old adage about "an ounce of prevention" takes on new meaning when it is applied to weight problems and diabetes. Prevention of type 2 diabetes literally saves lives.

Understanding the problem does not necessarily mean that a solution is at hand, however. Losing weight and maintaining a new "reduced" appearance is far from being a trivial task. The sheer number of books offering a "simple and quick" weight-loss plan tells me (and, it is hoped, you) that the problem is much more complex than these books imply. Otherwise, we would have solved the problem of obesity long ago. The truth is, there is no single recipe for weight loss. Weight maintenance requires a long-term commitment to a different (therapeutic) lifestyle.

Diabetes and obesity are two chronic conditions that cannot be cured or even controlled without the patient's active involvement. This book is meant to offer help to those who are ready and willing to get involved. My plan for weight loss and better health, which I've aptly named "the Draznin Plan," is based upon three principles: scientific facts, an individualized approach, and unwavering commitment to lifestyle changes. The lifestyle changes presented in this book will help you attain your goals—to improve or prevent type 2 diabetes and to maintain a healthy weight. However, only the combination of the Draznin Plan with your own personal commitment to my recommendations will bear the desired fruit. In other words, here I offer you a simple, easy-to-maintain plan for getting and staying healthier—actually following the plan will be up to you.

B. D.
Denver, Colorado
2003

# Contents

# Living with Diabetes

*Chapter One*

# At the Beginning

---

## A Letter to My Reader

When you took my book from the shelf in your favorite bookstore or library, you may have wondered what is so special about my program. In what way is Dr. Draznin's approach to weight loss and a healthier lifestyle better than dozens of others staring at you from the same bookshelf? What is the secret of the Draznin Plan that allows his patients to defeat their obesity and type 2 diabetes—the most common form of diabetes?

Not only do I encourage you to ask these questions, but also I hope you find convincing and reassuring answers in my book. I believe firmly that the more people understand about their weight problems and diabetes, the greater will be their commitment to improving their health, and the greater their chances for success. In most cases, weight maintenance and prevention of type 2 diabetes (which is frequently associated with

*I believe firmly that the more people understand about their weight problems and diabetes, the greater will be their commitment to improving their health, and the greater their chances for success.*

3

excess weight and insulin resistance—an inadequate action of insulin) are in the hands of patients themselves, and my role as a physician is simply to guide them through the often confusing obstacle course of energy *intake* (the number of calories we consume) and energy *expenditure* (the number of calories we burn).

Having treated thousands of patients with diabetes and obesity over more than three decades of academic medical practice, I have developed a unique program: the Draznin Plan. It is built on a solid scientific foundation, is easy to understand and follow, and has proven successful by patients who made a true commitment to their lifestyle changes.

The Draznin Plan is based on three principles—"a three-legged stool," if you will. The first is the science of clinical medicine, nowadays known as "evidence-based medicine." The cardinal feature of contemporary Western medicine is its reliance on controlled clinical studies to identify which treatments work and which do not. Anecdotal success stories, individual experiences with exotic therapies, and the popularity of non-traditional medical practices cannot substitute for the rigor of clinical research and scientific statistical analysis. Only proven therapies should be accepted as standards of care.

The field of weight maintenance is not an exception. Numerous clinical studies have repeatedly shown that any person on a low-calorie diet is going to lose weight. Interestingly, however, exercise without an accompanying diet failed to yield significant weight loss. Thus, telling patients that they can lose weight simply by increasing their energy expenditure would be misleading. In contrast, other studies have convincingly demonstrated that, after an initial weight loss, only those individuals who have incorporated exercise into their lifestyle have been able to maintain their reduced weight. The others regained their pounds. These studies are telling us that neither a low-calorie diet without exercise nor exercise without a low-calorie diet is adequate for long-term success in weight maintenance. This is why the combination of the Draznin Mile and the Draznin Calorie, which you'll learn about a little later on, works so effectively.

The second key principle (or leg in the "three-legged stool") of my approach is its individualized design. We are all distinct human beings, with our very own abilities to follow directions, maintain a program, and engage in physical activities. Each of us has his or her own tastes and food preferences, work schedule, lifestyle, and recreational interests. In a doctor's office, we expect an individualized approach to our medical problems. For example, I expect my physician to identify my problems specifically and to treat them accordingly. Otherwise, I could just walk into any pharmacy and buy over-the-counter medications to treat my maladies. Occasionally, we all do just that—but in most cases we want our doctors to do an examination, to find out why we cough, and to prescribe medications that are right for us. No two health problems are identical, even though many are alike. No two patients are the same either, even though they may have similar problems or symptoms. We should not settle for anything less in the treatment of obesity and diabetes.

The last and, unfortunately, weakest leg of this tripod is your own commitment to lifestyle changes, my dear reader. This is where most weight-loss programs fail. As the May 2002 issue of *Consumer Reports* stated, less than 25% of all dieters are able to keep their weight down for a year, regardless of the diet they use. Your ability to stick with the plan is integral to your success in losing weight and keeping it off.

The Draznin Plan is not a prescription for exercise. I am well aware that you are tired of being urged to exercise. I understand that you, my reader, cannot become an athlete or a spokesperson in a commercial for an exercise machine. Likewise, my approach does not consist of a set of recipes. The last thing you need is more recipes. Your bookshelf is already sagging under the weight of many cookbooks. You are a normal, living being—a reasonably active person who is not sweating in a gym or pedaling through miles of bike trails. You work, you take care of your home and your family, and you are mildly to moderately overweight. You wish to lose about 10 pounds and to drop one or two clothing sizes. You wish to get and stay healthy.

All of us—or, better said, almost all of us—with rare exceptions, love a hearty and tasty meal. Delicious and savory

*Eating should be a joy.* food is both pleasurable and fun. Eating should be a joy. Eating out is frequently an event. Good breakfast defines our day. A lovely picnic with friends provides lively entertainment. An elegant dinner is a wonderful nightcap. A diet, regardless of its composition, is seemingly an antonym of good living. A diet is a drag, a constant fight with guilt and frustration, a perpetual struggle. Why, then, do I recommend it to you? There is only one reason: to improve your health and, possibly, longevity. Only when you come to this very conclusion yourself will you be successful in maintaining a healthy diet, provided the diet offers variety, taste, and satiety.

My program will empower you to be in charge of your weight—and your diabetes, if you have it. It relies on simplicity, long-term goals, patience, and adjustments. Realistic expectations will become your guiding principles. I am confident that my down-to-earth concept will help you change your lifestyle forever.

Finally, here comes the most important question you might ask: Why should I buy your book, Dr. Draznin? Excellent question. And here is my four-point answer. First, and most important, my book offers practical, commonsense advice that will allow you to adopt the Draznin Plan into your daily life so as to achieve and maintain weight loss as well as to treat and prevent diabetes. Second, my book includes many real-life cases from my own practice (skillfully disguised, of course) that will aid you in your quest for meaningful lifestyle changes. Third, my book provides a scientific explanation, for those who wish to explore it, of how body weight is regulated and how we can therapeutically impact these regulatory mechanisms. Finally, this book was written by a world-renowned authority on diabetes and metabolic disorders, a professor of medicine at a major university, one of the leading diabetologists in the United States, and an author of many scientific articles, book chapters, and monographs in this field.

You, my reader, should now be ready to embark on a journey toward a very different lifestyle, and I (or my book, to be precise) will be your skipper, helping you maintain your new course. I offer what I believe is the most practical guide and the most realistic approach to your problems with weight maintenance. Over 100 of my own patients have used my plan and more than 80% of them achieved their goals. Will you be next?

Sincerely,
Boris Draznin, MD, PhD

## An Introductory Case

"I'm about fifty pounds overweight, I have high blood pressure, and my doctor told me I have a great deal of risk of developing diabetes," announced Mr. Jeffrey K. from his chair in my office. Jeff was six feet tall and weighed just over 230 lb. His shoulders slouched forward as he bent over his bulging belly. His left ankle rested over his right knee; this was because he could no longer cross his legs owing to a protruding stomach. "In short," he continued, after taking a deep breath, "I've been welcomed to the club. This is the first time in my life I have to actively resist joining a club—a club of obese diabetics. Can you help me?"

Jeff was wrong. He wasn't about to join this "exclusive" club—he had already joined it: a club of 28 million Americans who are overweight and 16 million Americans who have diabetes. His fasting blood-sugar level was 136 mg/dl (milligrams per deciliter), a full twenty-six points higher than the upper limit of the normal range, in the diagnostic criteria for diabetes. Normal fasting blood-sugar levels range between 70 and 110 mg/dl. Fasting blood-sugar levels greater than 126 mg/dl define diabetes. Levels between 110 and 126 mg/dl are designated as "impaired fasting glucose."

Jeffrey K. was a forty-seven-year-old successful lawyer, a "guru" in international business law, with strong entrepreneurial skills. He spoke fluent French and some German and spent about 60% of his time in Europe and Africa, attending to business deals. Hotel breakfast buffets, business lunches, and dinners had been his main diet for a number of years. Even at home he loved to take his family out to eat. He enjoyed ethnic foods and cold draft beer. The fact that he was gaining weight steadily was fairly obvious to him, but Jeff didn't like to think about it. A couple of times he had thought he should eat a bit less, but he loved his food so much that the very idea of dieting was simply foreign to him.

Jeff had never been very athletic, but in his college days he had loved to play touch football and softball. He even thought he was quite good at these sports, but he hadn't done anything in the way of exercise since his days at law school. He knew that many of the hotels where he stayed during his travels had health clubs, but he had never ventured out to any of them. He didn't feel like getting up early in the morning, and he was too tired, after a long working day, to exercise in the afternoon.

"Mr. K.," I replied, politely but firmly, "you do have diabetes. As you just pointed out, you also have obesity, the second largest preventable cause of premature death in this country. Only smoking causes more preventable deaths. There is a substantial probability that you can reverse your diabetes if you lose weight and return to a more active lifestyle. Not a guarantee, but you have a great chance for success.

"I have been doing research in diabetes and treating patients with diabetes and weight problems for more than thirty years," I continued. "These years of experience have allowed me to create and refine my own program, and it has helped many patients like yourself change their lifestyles, lose weight, and prevent the development of diabetes.

"You will have to eat less than you do now," I stressed, "and you will have to be much more active than you are now. I will teach you to exercise so that you will be able to walk up to three Draznin Miles a day and to eat up to eighteen Draznin Calories a day. I will also teach you where and what to eat when you dine out, how not to be hungry, and how to make physical activity a part of your life.

"The only way I can be of help to you, however, is if you and I reach a contract, which will require that you become an active participant in our efforts to restore your health. It won't be easy, and it won't be quick. You and I will have to introduce a lot of changes into your lifestyle, your attitude, and your commitment to health. I will guide you, but you will have to do the climbing to achieve our goal. I'll shed the light, but you'll have to walk the path. There are plenty of difficulties and frustrations along the way. You won't succeed unless you are totally dedicated to this goal. I cannot promise a cure, but, with your effort and commitment, we will certainly make significant improvement in your health and, consequently, longevity.

"Our success is in your hands," I concluded.

Jeff listened attentively, perhaps trying to guess what kinds of changes he would have to implement, how much frustration he would have to endure, how much commitment he would have to make, and how much trust he would have to put in me and my program.

"You are a successful businessman, Mr. K.," I continued, reading his thoughts in his expression. "The word 'failure' is not in your vocabulary. And the reason you don't fail is very simple: It is because of your commitment to your business, your adherence to your plans, your perseverance in pursuing your goals and objectives, your ability to take one step at a time, making adjustments as you move along, and your vision of the future. You and I both know that you have to possess these exceptional qualities to navigate in the business world. What we must do is apply the same qualities to your lifestyle, exactly as you have applied them to your business.

"I am going to offer you a set of rules. I don't know whether you will live longer if you follow the Draznin Rules, but I am certain that you'll increase your chances for longevity and undoubtedly enhance the quality of your life."

For several moments we sat in silence, looking straight into each other's eyes.

"You have three options," I said, with a smile, attempting to make it easier for Jeff. "You can leave this office right now and continue with your current lifestyle. You can spend an hour with me, hear my advice, and do with it whatever you wish. Take it or leave it, so to speak. Or you can decide to make a commitment to your own health and work with me to improve it."

Jeff pondered the options I offered him. We'll return to his reply later in the book. Meanwhile, let me tell you a little bit about myself and acquaint you with the Draznin Rules of life.

## The Origin of the Draznin Plan

My interest in diabetes may have been aroused by my own family history. My grandfather, my mother, and a maternal uncle had type 2 diabetes. For over thirty years, from the day I finished medical school, I have been doing clinical and basic research in the field of diabetes, studying insulin (one of the hormones that helps to regulate our weight) and how to achieve the best control

> *For over thirty years, from the day I finished medical school, I have been doing clinical and basic research in the field of diabetes, . . .*

over this chronic disease. I have also been trying to find the best dietary regimen for my patients. In the process, I have developed an approach to the problem of weight management that has been helpful to the majority of my patients.

I developed the concept of the Draznin Mile, in which the *duration* of activity, rather than the actual distance covered, is the measure of exercise. Later, I added the concept of the Draznin Calorie, in which any serving of food containing 100 calories is counted as one Draznin Calorie. Later in this book I will discuss the Draznin Mile and the Draznin Calorie in more detail so that you can begin to use these concepts in your own efforts to lose weight.

Using this system and a dozen Draznin Rules of lifestyle I've developed over the years, eight out of every ten of my patients were able to lose weight, keep it down, and prevent or get rid of their diabetes. This is an 80% success rate! Now I am ready to share my approach with anyone who wishes to lose weight and rid him- or herself of type 2 diabetes.

*Chapter Two*

# Our Weight in Numbers

---

*He who would eat the kernel must crack the nut.*

Danish proverb

The most amazing fact in the field of weight management is that the overwhelming majority of dieters in the United States do not need to lose weight, yet many people who do not need to lose weight are trying to do so. The culturally driven perception of "self-image" governs a widespread belief that we must be one or two clothing sizes smaller than we actually are. In contrast, only a small number of significantly overweight people—the ones who need to lose weight the most—are on diets.

This sounds like a paradox. Shouldn't it be the other way around? Shouldn't overweight people diet? The answer is yes, of course, but the fact remains—obese people are seldom on a diet. As we examine this apparent paradox a bit more carefully, we will see the depth of the problem. The discrepancy is easy to understand after we learn that 95% of those who lose weight on *any* diet regain it within the next twelve to twenty-four months. Not surprisingly, they give up on their diets. Frustration and denial replace drive and perseverance.

A survey conducted by *Consumer Reports* on the efficacy of various diets revealed that only 3% of participants had managed to complete formal weight-loss programs in the preceding three years. Even among those who had finished, the average success rate was only 26%. This is less than one-third of the 3% of people who began dieting in the first place! Demographically speaking, obese individuals as a group have lower incomes and less education than do nonobese people, and more frequently they remain single. The reasons for this are beyond the scope of this book, but it is clear that obesity has a high personal cost even before taking into account the adverse health consequences of being overweight.

## Ideal Body Weight and Body Mass Index

Because most of us in the United States (a virtual "land of plenty") carry an extra layer of subcutaneous fat, the question on everyone's mind is "How much is too much?" For years, the answer was relatively simple—if your weight was 20% greater than your ideal body weight, you were obese. With an answer like that, one must immediately ask the follow-up question, "What is the ideal body weight?"

The first attempt to define the ideal body weight came with the publication in 1959 of the Metropolitan Life Insurance Company tables. At that time, the tables demonstrated that the risk of premature death increased along with increased weight. The desirable weight, according to the Met Life tables, was 126 lb (57 kg) for a woman five feet four inches (1.63 cm) tall and 154 lb (70 kg) for a man five feet ten inches (1.78 cm) tall. Today, over 80% of the American public exceeds these standards.

If you are a man or woman of medium build, you can approximate, or "guesstimate," your ideal body weight. To do this, women should count 100 lb for the first five feet of their height. Then, they should add five pounds for each inch over five feet. For example, a five-foot six-inch woman would calculate her ideal body weight as 130 lb (100 lb for the first five feet and 5 lb × 6 = 30 lb for the additional six inches). Medium-built men should count 106 lb for the first five feet and add six pounds for each additional inch over five feet. A reasonable guesstimate of the ideal body weight for a six-foot man is 178 lb (106 lb for the first five feet and 6 lb × 12 = 72 lb for an additional twelve inches).

Subsequent studies showed that a ratio of weight to height (defined as weight in kilograms divided by the square of the height in meters) was a better surrogate for the risk of death from heart disease. This new ratio has come to be known as the body mass index, or BMI. For those of us who think in pounds and inches, the BMI can be calculated by dividing weight in pounds by height in inches squared and multiplying the quotient by 703. For example, a man who weighs 200 lb and is seventy inches tall has a BMI of 29: $(200 \div 70^2) \times 703 = (200 \div 4{,}900) \times 703 = 28.7$, or 29. Increases in BMI were found to be associated not only with heart disease but with many other health conditions also. Today's consensus (not without complications) is that a BMI greater than 27 confers a progressively increased risk of adverse health consequences (see Table 2.1).

*Obesity is clearly associated with diabetes, hypertension, heart disease, arthritis, and gallbladder disease, as well as cancer of the endometrium, breast, prostate, and colon.*

Obesity is clearly associated with diabetes, hypertension, heart disease, arthritis, and gallbladder disease, as well as cancer of the endometrium, breast, prostate, and colon.

**Table 2.1 BMI (kg/m$^2$) and the Risk of Death**

| BMI | Diagnostic Category |
| --- | --- |
| 19–25 | Normal weight |
| 26–29 | Overweight |
| 30–35 | Obese |
| 35–40 | Severely obese |
| Over 40 | Morbidly obese |

| Sex | BMI: Lowest Risk of Death |
| --- | --- |
| Men | 23.5–25 |
| Women | 22–23.5 |

Therefore, one way of defining the ideal body weight is to say that only a weight not associated with adverse health consequences is ideal. For practical purposes, this would be the weight that yields a BMI of less than 27.

A BMI of 19–25 is accepted as normal. Those of us with a BMI between 25 and 29 are considered overweight, and those with a BMI of over 30 are said to be obese. A BMI of 30–35 characterizes the moderately obese, a BMI between 35 and 40 defines severely obese people, and those with a BMI of over 40 are morbidly obese.

The first important caveat in using the BMI to define obesity is the fact that some very muscular and athletic people have high BMIs but no negative impact on their health. That is because their increased weight reflects the weight of strong muscles and not excess fat.

One of the best examples of the influence of muscle mass on the BMI was provided by Dr. Gary J. Davis, of Evanston Hospital, in a letter to the editor of the *New England Journal of Medicine*. Dr. Davis reported that basketball player Michael Jordan, by many accounts the athlete of the century, had a

BMI of 24, being 1.98 m tall and weighing 95 kg. This BMI placed Jordan on the less healthy end of the healthy-weight spectrum, although his body-fat content was under 10%. Even more striking, the body-fat content of another NBA star, Shaquille O'Neal, is reported to be approximately 5%, but his BMI is 29.7 (2.18 m height and 141 kg weight), placing him clearly in the obese category!

The second caveat is that at any given BMI individuals who are less fit have higher health risks than do their well-trained peers. In a study at the University of Alabama, researchers found that unfit but thin men with low BMIs—25 or lower—had twice the risk of death from all causes than did fit but overweight men with BMIs of 27.8 or greater. What this means is that the degree of muscle development and the state of fitness can greatly influence health risks outside the parameters of the BMI.

Finally, the distribution of fat in either the upper body (apple-shaped obesity) or the lower body (pear-shaped obesity) also confers different health risks, with upper-body obesity being more closely associated with adverse health consequences, such as heart disease, obesity, and hypertension. Upper-body obesity can be detected easily by measuring the circumference of the waist. People who are forty years old and younger with a waist circumference over forty inches and those over forty years old with a waist circumference greater than thirty-six inches have significantly increased cardiovascular risk.

## Obesity Rates Are Climbing

Around the world, both body weight and the prevalence of obesity are increasing rapidly. Epidemiologists, nutritionists, and diabetologists firmly believe that we now live in an era of epidemic obesity. The Worldwatch Institute, an Internet

**Table 2.2 Prevalence of Obesity**

| Group | Frequency of Obesity |
| --- | --- |
| U.S. adults | 55% Overweight |
|  | 22% Obese |
| U.S. children | 22% Boys obese |
|  | 25% Girls obese |
| European adults | 20% Overweight |

watchdog group, estimates that worldwide there are more obese than malnourished people. Today, 15%–20% of European adults and 50%–55% of Americans are significantly overweight (see Table 2.2).

The National Health and Nutrition Examination Surveys carried out by the National Center for Health Statistics have shown that 22.5% of the U.S. population is moderately to severely obese (BMI greater than 30), whereas some 55% of the total population is considered overweight (BMI greater than 27). This is a startling jump from the 14.1% obesity rate between 1971 and 1974 and the 14.5% rate between 1976 and 1980. Today, 63% of American men and 55% of American women have a BMI of 25 or higher, indicating that more than half of U.S. adults are considered either overweight or obese. More than 1.1 *billion* adults worldwide are overweight and 312 *million* of them are obese. According to the International Obesity Task Force (ironically, it exists), at least 155 million children worldwide are either obese or overweight.

A look at some more recent data, however, offers an even gloomier picture. Interestingly and sadly, the number of Americans who are about 100 lb or more overweight (this is a severely obese group, with a BMI of 40–50) grew by a staggering 50% between the years 2000 and 2005. This growth was twice as fast as in the group of people with moderate obesity (24%). But shockingly, the fastest-growing group was that of people with extreme obesity: the number of Americans with a BMI of 50 or higher increased by an incredible 75%!

When the risk of death from all causes together—or from cancer or heart disease separately—was calculated as a function of weight, it was found to increase substantially throughout the range of moderately to severely overweight individuals, both men and women, in all age groups. The lowest risk of death was found in men with a BMI of 23.5–25 and women with a BMI of 22–23.5. The relative risk of death remained low until the BMI exceeded 27 in men and 25 in women. In people with BMI values greater than these, the relative risk of death increased steadily.

Recently, the American Association of Retired Persons (AARP) issued a report on the health status of older Americans. It stated that even though "Americans over fifty are living longer, smoking less and developing fewer disabilities, increasing obesity could cancel the health gain." The report also states that between 1982 and 1999 obesity nearly doubled among those over age fifty, increasing from 14.4% to 26.7%.

Equally impressive is an increase in the prevalence of obesity among children. In boys aged six through eleven, the percentage of obesity increased from 15.2% to 22.3% between 1963 and 1991; for girls the percentage climbed from 15.8% to 22.7%. These numbers were steadily on the rise through the 1990s. Many pediatricians, pediatric endocrinologists,

*Many pediatricians, pediatric endocrinologists, and physicians working with adolescents have expressed genuine concern about the wave of obesity and even type 2 diabetes among children and young adults.*

and physicians working with adolescents have expressed genuine concern about the wave of obesity and even type 2 diabetes among children and young adults. As recently as ten to fifteen years ago, type 2 diabetes was exceptionally rare, almost unheard of, in children and adolescents. The epidemic of obesity has changed this reality and introduced type 2 diabetes to a generation of our children.

## Why Are We Becoming More Obese?

The reason or, more appropriately, reasons for the dramatic increase in the prevalence of obesity are not completely clear. I cannot offer you a definitive answer—entire books have been written on this subject, and researchers are still trying to puzzle out the complexities of this problem. What we do know is that obesity has a relatively strong genetic component—meaning we inherit some of the risk for obesity from our parents—even though the genes responsible for this specific obesity-prone background have not yet been identified.

However, the rapid progression of this epidemic cannot be explained by genetic influence alone. There is no reason to believe that there has been a recent major change in the genetic makeup of inhabitants of the Western world. We can assume that the propensity for obesity—the genes that predispose us to store energy and gain weight—must have been with us for generations. Recent changes in environmental factors must have had a huge impact in order for the incidence of obesity to explode as it has. To prove this point, let's consider the Amish. Obesity among Amish children is rare. A recent study compared the prevalence of obesity and the levels of physical activity in children from a rural Old Order Amish community with children living in modern society. Researchers found that only 7% of the Amish children were overweight and only 1.4%

were obese. Among non-Amish American and Canadian children of the same age, 25% were overweight and up to 9.5% of boys and 11.7% of girls were obese. The activity logs kept by the Amish children indicated that they performed multiple daily chores requiring considerable physical activity. They milked cows, gardened, fed farm animals, and carried wood. What's more, most Amish children walk to school regardless of weather conditions. What this study tells us is that physical activity has an enormous impact on obesity.

Physical activity is only half of the story. Our lifestyles have become more and more sedentary, yes. But the increase in availability of food, particularly of high–caloric density items, constitutes another important change our society has experienced in the last two to three decades.

I would like to draw your attention to an interesting relationship between the rise in obesity rates in the last fifteen years or so and historical changes in nutritional recommendations in the United States. In 1921, it was recommended that we consume 20% of our daily ration in the form of carbohydrate. This figure gradually increased to 40% in the 1950s and to 45% in the 1970s. In the 1970s and early 1980s, there was a tendency among nutritionists and diabetologists to consider carbohydrates, especially refined sugars, "pure, white, and deadly." Such was the title of the book published by a British diabetologist, Dr. J. Yudkin, in 1986. Since then, the perceptions of nutritionists and their attitudes toward carbohydrates have changed dramatically. Suddenly, around 1985 or 1986, American nutritionists began advocating 60% carbohydrate in a healthy diet! What we called the "prudent" diet of the 1990s recommended that the food we eat contain 50%–55% carbohydrate. Even though one cannot draw any solid conclusions about a cause-and-effect relationship, a distinct parallel exists between the jump in carbohydrate consumption and the rise in obesity. Why did the experts in nutrition increase their advocacy for carbohydrates? They did not mean to harm us. They did not wish to worsen the epidemic of obesity in this country. They recommended what they saw as the best eating strategy for a healthy lifestyle at that time. And yet they have created a problem that will take years to undo.

First of all, in my experience, most of the well-meaning specialists in nutrition are also committed to strenuous exercise and heavy-duty workouts. They bike and run, and they fill aerobic classes to capacity. They are constantly engaged in recreational activities and proudly display to the rest of us their slim, muscular bodies, dressed in sweat-drenched athletic attire. They need tons of extra energy to cover the expenditure that occurs during exercise, and they find this readily available energy in high-carbohydrate food. They became and remain completely oblivious to the fact that most of us do not exercise at all! They have blanketed us with the message of the benefit of a high-carbohydrate diet, forgetting a simple truth: What's sauce for the goose is not always sauce for the gander.

While nutritionists and exercise enthusiasts were promoting their love for the high-carbohydrate diet, scientists began to understand that cholesterol and other fats might have a detrimental effect on the heart and blood vessels. At the beginning, no distinction was made between "bad" fat and "good" fat, between the "Western" diet and the "Mediterranean" diet, or between the influences of saturated and unsaturated fats. Fat in the diet became synonymous with a death sentence. This grew to the point where some parents withheld milk from their children in their zeal to eliminate fat from their offspring's diets. The food industry, willingly or unwillingly, was also dragged into this craze. "Low-fat" and "no-fat" items filled the shelves of supermarkets. The problem was that all that "nasty" fat was being replaced by huge amounts of carbohydrates! Elimination of fatty foods and reduction in fat content might have had a beneficial effect, as this would have reduced the total number of calories consumed, but not when all those calories were simply replaced by carbohydrates.

Poor reasoning inadvertently killed the good deed, much like the proverbial road to hell that is paved with good intentions. Many food items, particularly those that contain hefty doses of carbohydrates, proudly display the "Food Guide Pyramid" on their labels. The base of the pyramid represents bread, cereal, rice, and pasta—food choices recommended by the guide. For a sedentary individual, this pyramid is not an ancient wonder but the best prescription to promote obesity!

## Obesity and Its Relationship with Diabetes

Obesity is not a trivial or innocent condition. Approximately 300,000 Americans die every year from complications attributable to obesity. These complications constitute the second leading cause of preventable death in America, after complications from smoking. It is now estimated that one-third of all people born after the year 2000 will develop diabetes at some point in their lives.

*Approximately 300,000 Americans die every year from complications attributable to obesity.*

One of the most common conditions that accompanies obesity is type 2 diabetes. Obviously, not all overweight or even severely obese individuals develop diabetes, but the risk for the disease substantially increases with weight. Not surprisingly, both incidence (the number of new cases in a given time period) and prevalence (the total number of cases in a given population) of diabetes increase in parallel with increasing rates of obesity. The relative risk of developing diabetes in individuals with a BMI of 24–25 is about 5%. The risk doubles, growing to 10%, in those with a BMI of 27–29 and quadruples (to 20%) in those with a BMI of 29–31. The risk escalates further to 40% in people with a BMI of 33–35 and to an incredible 60% in individuals with a BMI greater than 35. Conversely, statistics show that over 85% of patients with type 2 diabetes are obese. Each year, approximately 800,000 Americans are diagnosed with the condition. About 90% of these, or 720,000, have type 2 diabetes. If 85% of these newly diagnosed individuals are obese, the country will acquire 612,000 patients with diabetes and obesity annually.

A slightly higher number of women have diabetes than men, and the incidence of diabetes increases with age. On average, African Americans and Latino/Hispanic Americans are almost twice as likely to have diabetes as are Caucasians of similar age. We don't know exactly why this is, although the reason most likely has to do with genetic differences between ethnicities. It is estimated that, in the United States, approximately 25% of all adult patients with type 2 diabetes belong to minority groups.

The rate of death—from any cause—among middle-aged people with diabetes is twice as high as that for middle-aged people without diabetes. For example, the relative risk of heart attack is 50% greater in diabetic men and 150% greater in diabetic women than in their nondiabetic counterparts. Diabetic men are 50% more likely to die suddenly (sudden death is mainly due to heart attack or stroke) than men in the general population. For women, the disparity is even greater, with sudden death being 300% more common in diabetic than in nondiabetic ones.

Both obesity and diabetes are closely associated with heart disease, mainly atherosclerotic coronary artery disease, which can lead to heart attacks, chest pain (angina), and stroke. Problems with atherosclerosis in patients with diabetes and/or obesity begin with what is called "inflammation" in the blood vessel walls. This inflammation is marked by the appearance of a protein called C-reactive protein (CRP). The greater the inflammation, the more CRP is found in the blood. Recent studies indicate that consumption of food items with high concentrations of rapidly absorbed carbohydrates results in substantial increases in the appearance of CRP in blood in apparently healthy middle-aged women. These findings suggest that intake of such foods may increase the risk not only of diabetes but of atherosclerosis and heart disease.

Poorly controlled diabetes triggers numerous other complications and medical problems. Almost half of new cases of end-stage kidney failure leading to either dialysis or kidney transplantation are related to diabetes. Most patients with diabetes suffer nerve damage after fifteen to twenty years with the disease. Diabetes is also a leading cause of nontraumatic leg amputation (82,000 cases in 2002, according to the Centers for Disease Control and Prevention, www.cdc.gov), and approximately 20% of male patients with diabetes complain of impotence. In the United States, diabetes is a leading cause of new cases of blindness among people twenty to seventy-five years of age; in 2002, there were 24,000 new cases of blindness attributable to diabetes. Eye disease, particularly problems with small blood vessels of the background of the eye (known as the retina), is a very common complication of diabetes. These little conduits of blood can grow uncontrollably and break, causing retinal detachment and severe bleeding inside the eye. Increased fluid pressure within the eye (glaucoma) and damage to the optic nerve (the main nerve of the eye that transmits the image from the retina to the brain) can also occur with increased frequency in diabetes.

It is not surprising that a problem of such magnitude is on the minds of thousands of Americans who are eager and almost ready to turn the tide of obesity in this country. That's where this book comes in. In the chapters that follow, you will be introduced to the details of the Draznin Plan, along with the guidance and information you will need to implement my weight-loss strategies, to avoid the dangers of obesity, and to prevent (or treat) diabetes.

*In the chapters that follow, you will be introduced to the details of the Draznin Plan...*

## Chapter Three

# The Law of Conservation of Energy

D espite amazing advances in the biomedical sciences, physicians and scientists do not really know why some of us gain weight so easily while others eat just about everything they see (the "see-food diet"—you see food, you eat it!) and remain slim. We also have very little information about why some of us overweight creatures develop diabetes while others, equally overweight, do not. Much of the reason is probably genetic, our vulnerability to obesity and diabetes determined by the genes we have inherited from our parents.

Therefore, the first Draznin Rule is as follows: The most important step in life is to choose your parents correctly. If one were to follow this rule (and it isn't easy!) and do it well, the rest would simply fall into place. One would neither be over-

*. . . the first Draznin Rule is as follows: The most important step in life is to choose your parents correctly.*

weight nor develop diabetes. However, the genes that determine whether we are destined to become overweight seem to be extremely prevalent and to occur with great frequency. It is safe to say that the majority of us, given unlimited access to food, have a tendency to gain weight.

Centuries ago, when our food supply was erratic and predictably unpredictable, the genes that allowed our ancestors to store more fat, and thereby more energy, were beneficial to our survival and, as such, spread among the population. Today, in a time of plenty, these genes are more than just a nuisance and we have to fight their fat-storing influence on an almost daily basis.

## Energy Consumption and Expenditure

Energy is the most fundamental requirement for all aspects of life. For any biological process to occur, an organism, whether it is a single-cell alga or a complex mammal, must possess enough energy to cover the demands of this process. The very survival of the organism depends on finding and acquiring appropriate quantities of energy to sustain life. However, if an organism acquires more energy than is necessary to cover its needs, excess energy is stored within the body and used appropriately when new energy intake is limited.

Let us digress for a moment and examine what determines our ability to accumulate fat. Most of us have heard about the law of conservation of energy (even though just a few of us truly understand it):

$$energy\ we\ consume = energy\ we\ expend$$

If we consume more energy than we expend, excess energy will be retained and stored by the body, and the equation will look like this:

$$energy\ we\ consume - energy\ we\ expend$$
$$= energy\ we\ retain$$

The energy we expend consists of three parts: the basal metabolic rate, the energy we expend to support physical activities, and the energy we expend to support miscellaneous functions of the body (we don't really know where it

*The basal metabolic rate, or BMR . . . is the amount of energy required to support the work of the heart, brain, lungs, and other organs at rest, in the absence of any physical or mental exertion.*

all goes). The *basal metabolic rate*, or BMR (also known as *resting energy expenditure*), is the amount of energy required to support the work of the heart, brain, lungs, and other organs at rest, in the absence of any physical or mental exertion. The BMR accounts for approximately 50%–65% of our total daily energy expenditure. The energy we expend on physical activity is called *activity thermogenesis,* or AT (also known as *voluntary energy expenditure*), while the third component of energy expenditure is known as *non-exercise-associated thermogenesis*, or NEAT, the amount of energy we spend fidgeting.

Finally, a small amount of energy is spent on breaking down (digesting) and absorbing food, the biochemical conversion of nutrients during the metabolic cycle, and the production of new energy.

This looks like an investment in a process that generates much more energy in return. This expenditure is called the *thermic effect of food,* or TE, and it accounts for about 10% of the total daily energy expenditure. Therefore:

$$calories\ consumed = BMR + AT + NEAT + TE$$

(The term "calorie," as used in this book, represents 1,000 calories or 1 kilocalorie [1 kcal]. See Chapter 10 for the scientific definition of "calorie.") Again, if we expend less than we consume, the remaining energy will be stored:

$$calories\ consumed = BMR + AT + NEAT + TE$$
$$+ calories\ in\ storage\ (weight\ gain)$$

Conversely, if we expend more than we consume, we will lose energy from storage and lose weight:

$$BMR + AT + NEAT + TE - calories\ consumed$$
$$= calories\ removed\ from\ storage\ (weight\ loss)$$

With food being the only energy source for creatures like us, the mouth is the only loading dock for delivering energy supplies to the body. We know that "man does not live by bread alone," and yet food is our only source of energy. If we expend almost all the energy we consume, very little will be left over to store. In other words, the energy that remains in the body at the end of the day is the difference between the energy we have obtained from food and the energy we have spent during that day. Roughly, each time the amount of energy consumed exceeds the amount of energy spent by approximately 3,500 calories, we gain one pound of fat. This means that just a little over 500 calories per day in extra food will be converted into a pound of fat in a week. This equation, 3,500 calories = 1 lb of fat, is important to remember not only because of its negative connotation but also for your future success in losing weight. A deficit of 3,500 calories will result in a one-pound weight loss.

The second Draznin Rule is as follows: If longevity is in your genes, the quality of your life is in your hands. Predisposition to type 2 diabetes is defined by the genes we inherit from our parents. Some of these genes

*The second Draznin Rule is as follows: If longevity is in your genes, the quality of your life is in your hands.*

remain silent until environmental influence, such as weight gain, reveals their presence. For example, as I gain weight and become more and more insulin-resistant, my pancreas must produce more and more insulin to overcome the resistance to this hormone my body builds. However, my pancreas is genetically programmed to produce only a certain amount of insulin and cannot keep up with the demands imposed by my weight gain. Because of these genetic limitations, at a certain point my pancreas will no longer be able to meet the demands and my predisposition to diabetes will convert into overt disease.

## How Calories Are Absorbed (or Not)

The law of conservation of energy is indisputable, unshaken by any doubts, and it remains the basis for our understanding of weight gain and weight loss. But the law comes with caveats. Nothing in life is as simple as it appears to be. First, not all the food that enters our mouths is consumed by our bodies and utilized as calories. Some of this food is never absorbed. It passes through the gastrointestinal tract and is expelled at the other end. Let us assume that two individuals, Mr. A. and Mr. B., have each eaten a bowl of cereal containing 300 calories of energy. That day, Mr. A. had diarrhea. We do not know at this point why he received an urgent call to the bathroom—maybe he just returned from a trip to a foreign country (traveler's diarrhea), or maybe he had lactose intolerance or some other medical problem. Regardless of the cause of his diarrhea, he will absorb only part of the 300 calories he consumed. He will certainly have consumed fewer calories than Mr. B., who has no gastrointestinal problems. Now, this is an extreme example— in real life, there is a spectrum of levels of food absorption among people aside from that caused by diarrhea or constipation. Variations are numerous. Chances are good that you and your spouse, for example, do not absorb exactly the same numbers of calories, even after eating exactly the same meal. This is just a fact of life that arises from our distinct genetic makeup and body composition.

The second important variable in food absorption stems from the fact that certain foods are absorbed much better and faster than others. For example, a teaspoon of sugar is absorbed almost instantaneously, whereas a teaspoon of pasta requires significantly more time for digestion. The complex carbohydrates of pasta must first be broken down by the digestive system into simple sugars; then they are absorbed. In contrast, each molecule of table sugar consists of only two simple sugars that are readily absorbed. It is not surprising then that we absorb 8 oz of ice cream much faster than 8 oz of filet mignon.

Recently, new therapeutic strategies have been developed in an attempt to modulate food absorption, and thereby influence caloric consumption. The class of drugs called "alpha-glucosidase inhibitors" blocks the breakdown of complex carbohydrates into simple sugars. Complex carbohydrates are not absorbed in the small intestine but instead moved down through the intestine to be evacuated. If you were to eat a plate of pasta while taking these drugs, only a portion of what you ate would be absorbed. A great deal of your pasta would escape breakdown and absorption and would be eliminated. Similarly, the drug orlistat blocks the activities of enzymes that help absorb dietary fats. Therefore, when you take orlistat, only a fraction of the dietary fat that found its way into your mouth will be absorbed (and, consequently, stored by the body).

This pharmacological tinkering with natural absorption is not without side effects. When carbohydrate breakdown in the small intestine is impaired by drugs, the carbohydrates move to the large intestine, where local microbes, which love to decompose carbohydrates, have a field day. While the microbes proliferate and digest as many carbohydrate molecules as they can find, they also create a lot of gas in the large intestine. Gas has a natural way of escaping, which may place a person taking these drugs in an untenable position. Furthermore, since orlistat blocks fat absorption, unabsorbed fat may slide down into the large intestine; it may even leak out of the body, often uncontrollably. These side effects are usually minor and create only minimal inconvenience, but occasionally they can push a person into social isolation.

## How Calories Are Utilized (or Not)

Absorption and consumption of calories differ among individuals; what's more, once these calories are absorbed, their utilization can vary dramatically from person to person. Let us return to our friends Mr. A. and Mr. B. Mr. A.'s diarrhea has now passed, and he and Mr. B. each eat two slices of pizza, about 700 calories per piece, for a total of 1,400 calories.

By the time they finish, it is about 10:00 PM. Mr. A. and Mr. B. are equally physically active. They both go to sleep. Their bodies use the newly acquired energy to support their breathing, food digestion, heart and brain activity, urine production (all these bodily systems work on, even as they sleep), and occasional movement during the night (turning and tossing in bed). Their bodies expend a sizable amount of energy to cover their basic metabolic needs, the BMR. It turns out that because of differences in their genetic makeup, these two men have very different BMRs. Metabolically speaking, Mr. A.'s body is extremely efficient. He requires half the energy that Mr. B. requires to support his metabolic needs. While he is asleep, his body uses only 800 calories, leaving 600 calories (1,400 calories – 800 calories = 600 calories) for storage and

future use. In contrast, Mr. B.'s body is exceptionally inefficient, and he has had to use 1,100 calories to support his basic
metabolic needs. This means that he has only 300 calories left
for storage and future use (1,400 calories − 1,100 calories =
300 calories).

Not surprisingly, Mr. B. will not gain as much weight as Mr.
A., even though they both ate exactly the same amount. When
they wake up and go to the local health club to work out, they
will discover an interesting detail. In the absence of physical
activity, Mr. A. burns fewer calories than does Mr. B. Therefore, Mr. A. will have to exercise almost twice as much as Mr. B.
in order to reduce to the same degree the amount of energy he
stores.

### Insulin Levels and Activity

There is one more important concept that Mr. A. and Mr. B.
(and the rest of us) should know about when considering
"individualized" ways of utilizing calories. The way our calories
are directed to either storage or utilization is under the constant
and rigorous control of *insulin,* a hormone responsible for the maintenance of normal levels of glucose (blood sugar) in the blood. The activity
and levels of this hor-
mone, as well as its abil-
ity to work, are critically important for the utilization of
glucose by muscles and fat, for energy storage in both the liver
and muscle, and for the growth and development of new and
old fat cells in the body.

*The way our calories are directed to either storage or utilization is under the constant and rigorous control of insulin, a hormone responsible for the maintenance of normal levels of glucose (blood sugar) in the blood.*

The latter is particularly important to understand. One cannot accumulate fat and become overweight in the absence of insulin. People who develop insulin deficiency, so-called type 1 diabetes, lose weight very rapidly in a process called *lipolysis,* which is an accelerated breakdown of fat cells. We will return to insulin later in this book, but for now it will suffice to say that both the levels and the activity of insulin represent the third important variable that modifies the law of conservation of energy in the human body.

*Chapter Four*

# The Draznin Mile: A New Concept of Exercise

---

I t is no secret that most of us do not like to exercise. Hence, the third Draznin Rule is as follows: Desire to exercise

*. . . the third Draznin Rule is as follows: Desire to exercise is inversely proportional to age.*

is inversely proportional to age. Healthy preschoolers, almost without exception, are remarkably active. Chasing your three- or four-year-old offspring can be an exhausting full-time job. By the end of grade school, however, the vast majority of children stop running, skipping, and jumping. The average American child now spends three hours a day in front of the TV set and at least one and a half hours a day in front of the computer. In junior high school, physical education class is considered boring by at least 75% of students. At the same time, four basic food groups emerge as the staple diet of teenagers: fast food, soft drinks, candy, and sugar-coated cereals.

By the age of thirty, only a tiny minority of individuals engage in regular exercise. For those over thirty, sport is now a spectacle—something we view from a chair, a sofa, or bleachers. At the age of forty, we enter a period of life known as "middle age." (By the way, "middle age" is best defined as your own age, dear reader, and younger.) In addition to the plethora of well-described peculiarities attributed to middle-age crises, many middle-aged men and women make a feeble attempt to return to an active lifestyle. This attempt is almost never successful and rarely lasts longer than a year. A notable exception is the good tennis player. Tennis players tend to stay active longer, usually until their knees can no longer take the abuse. Golfers who classify their game as exercise, particularly those who drive electric carts, indulge in self-deception.

For most of us, it is much more pleasant to lie by the pool with a good book in our hands (after a quick five- to ten-minute dip) than to swim multiple laps for an hour. In my neighborhood, over 80% of the houses have a basketball hoop, but in the last five years I have not seen a single neighbor over forty shooting hoops! I have seen a few of my forty-plus neighbors jog. But the grimaces on their faces as they return home reveal both the misery and the displeasure caused by this form of exercise. Recently, biking, particularly family bicycling, has come into vogue. For a while, I felt very encouraged by seeing a family of four or five on the bike path, but it appears that most people give up biking as a form of exercise as soon as their teenage children stop riding with them. The truth of the matter is that, unlike competitive sports, where the goal is to be first (by definition, the strongest and the best), exercise for the sake of sweating, in the name of longevity, is simply contrary to human nature.

Having said all this, I wish to proclaim that exercise is the single most important element for living a healthy life. The right amount of physical activity makes us feel better, helps keep weight down, supports our aging backs, allows for better circulation, and beefs up our ability to cope with stress. The question is, how can we incorporate the right amount of exercise into our lives, into our daily routines? How can exercise become one of the basic activities of daily living, such as bathing, dressing, eating, and so forth? If we who have an inherited aversion to exercise could only find a way of making exercise an integral part of our lives, we would lose weight, reduce blood pressure, remove at least 80% of our tension and anxiety, defeat diabetes (in most cases), live longer, and feel better.

## Understanding the Draznin Mile

Years of searching for a "magic recipe" for exercise have finally paid off with the invention of the Draznin Mile. Here is my formula: Walk three to four Draznin Miles each day, or jog three Draznin Miles every other day. The Draznin Mile is the simplest way to measure your exercise. What is a Draznin Mile, you ask? Here's how it works: The Draznin Mile defines the duration of your exercise—not the distance, and certainly not the speed. Ten minutes of jogging or twenty minutes of walking equals one Draznin Mile. If you have jogged for ten minutes, you can call it a Draznin Mile. If you have jogged for twenty minutes, you have done two Draznin Miles, no matter what the actual distance was. The distance is totally irrelevant. Never, never, never worry about the distance. *The time is what is important.*

If it so happens that you have, indeed, jogged one mile in ten minutes, you are doing much better than expected. A ten-minute mile means that you can cover six miles in an hour. Please, never even think of doing that! You don't need it. No one needs it. All you need to do is three Draznin Miles, meaning a thirty-minute jog. If your weight is 175 lb, with a jogging speed of ten minutes per mile, you will burn eleven calories per minute, or 330 calories in thirty minutes.

Do you see how easy it gets? If you jog two Draznin Miles, you burn 220 calories. In real life, however, for ordinary people like you and me the speed is totally irrelevant. Thus, the fourth Draznin Rule is as follows: A ten-minute jog covers one Draznin Mile and burns 110 calories. I recommend that

*... the fourth Draznin Rule is as follows: A ten-minute jog covers one Draznin Mile and burns 110 calories.*

you jog at least three Draznin Miles every other day. Doing that, you will burn 330 calories every other day, or about 1,000–1,200 calories per week.

There are two things I want you to keep in mind, however. The first is the intensity of exercise. Intensity level is not important at all when you first embark on my program. In the beginning, the most important point is to engrave a habit of exercising firmly into your daily life. At this stage, the critical element of my program is to incorporate physical activity into a new lifestyle. Later on, the intensity will become a significant issue to consider.

Low-intensity exercise is basically equivalent to the basal metabolic rate (BMR) in terms of energy expenditure. This is why light gardening and cooking do not help in losing weight. One is active all right, but the intensity of the activity is too low to burn excess energy. The intensity of exercise must be at least moderate so as to expend energy over and above the BMR. Exercise physiologists call this "exercise at 65% or 75% of maximal capacity, determined by your heart rate and oxygen consumption." I can assure you, however, that if you do three Draznin Miles a day, at least five days a week, you will reach the necessary intensity to achieve your goal.

The second thing to keep in mind is your gender. I guess that rarely escapes our minds. What I really mean is that there is a significant gender-dependent difference in energy expenditure, particularly at the tender ages of fifty-five and over. In order to burn 300 calories, a sixty-five-year-old man must exercise for approximately forty minutes. In contrast, a sixty-five-year-old woman may have to exercise for seventy minutes to burn the same 300 calories. Whether or not this difference is related to loss of estrogen function during menopause is unknown, but the fact remains—women must exercise longer, at the same level of intensity, to burn the same number of calories as men do.

Now, what if you cannot jog? Not to worry. This is just fine. The Draznin walking mile is what you cover during a twenty-minute walk. In other words, if you have walked for twenty minutes, you have covered a mile. Your actual speed (if you indeed were to cover one mile in twenty minutes) would be three miles per hour, or half a mile in ten minutes. At that speed, you burn 5.55 calories per minute. But, as with jogging, the actual distance is irrelevant. The Draznin Mile is a twenty-minute walk, so if you walk for forty minutes, you have done two Draznin walking-miles and burned 220 calories. Not bad! After a sixty-minute walk, you will have lost 330 calories. The fifth Draznin Rule is as follows: A twenty-minute walk covers one mile and burns 110 calories. It is easy to see that, if you jog or walk a Draznin Mile (ten or twenty minutes, respectively), you will lose approximately 110 calories.

*The fifth Draznin Rule is as follows: A twenty-minute walk covers one mile and burns 110 calories.*

I recommend that you walk for sixty minutes, at least five days a week. You can do it in one walk or split it into two sessions: a walk in the morning and one in the evening. Your goal is to do three Draznin Miles every other day if you are a jogger or three to four Draznin Miles every day if you prefer to walk. Then, when you talk with your friends or relatives or colleagues, you can proudly say that you are doing three or four Draznin Miles either every day or every other day. They will be duly impressed, and you will truly be doing a great favor for yourself.

## Getting Started

This is your goal, but you should start on a much smaller scale. Common sense never hurts. As far as I am concerned, common sense dictates starting with a short five-minute walk. Just stroll out of your house and walk for five minutes along the straightest segment of the road in front of your dwelling. Walk five minutes by your watch. That would certainly mean that you would need another five minutes to return home. So take a deep breath and continue toward home. Congratulations! You have just done a ten-minute walk and covered half a Draznin Mile. (If you cannot walk for five minutes in each direction, you have a serious problem. This book is unlikely to help at this stage.)

Remember that your goal is to walk three to four Draznin Miles. You are not that far off. By the second week you should increase the time you walk in each direction to ten minutes, for a total of twenty minutes of walking—and that is a Draznin Mile! This is what you should do for the entire week. Increase the amount of time you walk by two minutes per week and, five weeks later, you will be walking two Draznin Miles a day, or twenty minutes, equal to one Draznin Mile, in each direction. Do that for an entire month. Do not skip a single day. I want you to do a month of two Draznin Miles per day. In so doing, you will expend 220 calories a day in addition to your normal daily energy expenditure.

At the end of the month you will have two options: You can continue increasing your walking time (and distance) by two minutes a week until you are doing three Draznin Miles per day, or you can start walking in the evening (before or after dinner) and build your evening walk up to one or two Draznin Miles.

Some of my patients have honestly complained, and not without reason, that walking is inordinately boring. Fifteen or twenty minutes might be okay, but anything beyond twenty to twenty-five minutes becomes a difficult chore. Fortunately, electronic engineers have invented the Walkman, the Discman, the iPod, and other listening devices that are exceptionally helpful in this regard. Just turn on your favorite radio program or CD or cue up your favorite play list and begin your march. Instead of listening from your couch to the click and clack of National Public Radio, put on your earphones and go for an hour's walk while still enjoying your favorite recording artist or composer. You will find that the boredom of walking will vanish with the first musical chords. I even have patients who listen to books on tape while walking. I just hope this does not replace their reading hour!

By the way, if you decide to use a treadmill at home, consider placing it in front of a TV set. Most of my patients watch TV at least thirty minutes a day, being addicted to the local and national news, various news-related programs, and other shows. I recommend that they watch TV while walking a couple of Draznin Miles, and many do. I must admit—I do it myself! If you opt for jogging and have never exercised before, you should start with a two-minute jog each way. Even though it sounds like nothing, this is the best way to get into the routine. As we walking, you should add two minutes of jogging in each direction every week until you are jogging three Draznin Miles comfortably every other day. Congratulations, once again—you have reached your goal!

## Finding Alternative Forms of Exercise

Before we end this chapter, there is one more point to discuss. One day I spent a full hour outlining an exercise program for a patient, Ms. J., only to learn, at the end of our conversation, that she cannot walk! She had had frequent dislocations of her ankle and could not really undertake the risk of daily walking.

So we turned to alternatives. The first alternative is swimming. It is a lovely form of exercise for good swimmers. Unfortunately, I have found that, for most of us, it is not a good option. There is not enough muscular work in leisurely, noncompetitive swimming. Most people get tired because of labored breathing long before their muscles have expended sufficient amounts of energy. But if swimming is your only option, a twenty-minute swim equals one Draznin Mile. Three Draznin Miles every other day is all you need! The second alternative is bicycling. This form of exercise is much better, but one must use a stationary bike and not a street bike. Not all of us feel comfortable on a street bike; this is true not only on the street but even along bike paths. As a rule, people who are significantly overweight do not have the agility necessary to ride a bike. Finally, bike riding carries an inherent danger of falling, which is better avoided. The problem with either a street bike or a stationary one is that riding without resistance is very inefficient in terms of burning energy. One has to spend much more time on a bike to achieve the level of energy expenditure that one would attain per unit of time jogging. Therefore, if you must be on a bike, thirty minutes of nonstop pedaling without resistance equals one Draznin Mile. To do three Draznin Miles, you will have to pedal for ninety minutes. However, that can be rather boring. One can increase the effectiveness of bicycling by either choosing programs with more resistance or doing uphill rides. In any event, biking can be a viable alternative to jogging or walking (Table 4.1).

A word of caution for those who are actually preparing to buy new walking shoes: Anyone over the age of thirty-five or who might have a medical condition, particularly a heart problem, must undergo a stress test before embarking on an exercise program. Your primary care physician can refer you to a specialist to perform this test. This is a simple but extremely important precaution that should not be overlooked.

*Anyone over the age of thirty-five or who might have a medical condition, particularly a heart problem, must undergo a stress test before embarking on an exercise program.*

People who have already developed complications of diabetes should be extremely careful with their exercise regimen. This is particularly true for those with diabetic retinopathy (problems with the blood vessels at the back of the eye), kidney

**Table 4.1 Draznin Mile Equivalents**

One Draznin Mile equals
1. 10 min jogging or
2. 20 min walking or
3. 20 min swimming or
4. 30 min biking without resistance
and burns approximately 110 calories. Three Draznin Miles a day will allow one to burn 330 calories.

disease, and heart conditions. They should not be doing weight lifting, jogging, or boxing. Walking and swimming are the most appropriate forms of exercise for these individuals. Assuming you have none of these problems, within four to six months you should make three Draznin Miles your daily routine.

## Chapter Five

# Insulin, Production and Storage of Energy, and Regulation of Weight

I believe a little dose of science is in order at this point. I subscribe to the theory that the more people understand about their medical conditions and the way their bodies work, the greater the chances for successful therapeutic interventions. This is particularly applicable to the health problems that require lifestyle changes. Having said this, I acknowledge readily that not everyone is interested in the science underlying his or her medical problems. I would not be affronted at all if you decide to skip this chapter entirely or return to it later, after finishing the rest of the book (I hope you'll do the latter). This chapter is here to make the scientific background of insulin, energy, and regulation of weight available to those who wish to learn more.

*This chapter is here to make the scientific background of insulin, energy, and regulation of weight available to those who wish to learn more.*

Insulin is undoubtedly one of the most important hormones in the human body. A protein produced in the pancreas, a gland located in the upper part of the abdomen, insulin is released into the bloodstream in response to sugar. Without insulin, a person usually cannot survive more than a couple of weeks—seldom as long as a couple of months. This condition of complete, or almost complete, lack of insulin is known as *type 1 diabetes mellitus.* The only hormone in the body that reduces blood-sugar levels, insulin

- Is produced in the pancreas
- Is released in response to meals
- Stimulates utilization and storage of sugars
- Stimulates formation of new fat and proteins
- Prevents breakdown of fat and proteins
- Is absolutely required for survival

Type 1 diabetes most commonly occurs in children and young adults (hence, it was formerly known as "juvenile-onset diabetes"), but it can appear at any age. It is believed to be an autoimmune disease, wherein an unknown trigger commands the body to destroy its own insulin-producing cells. Synthetic insulin is a life-saving treatment for patients with type 1 diabetes.

When we ingest carbohydrates, they are broken down into simple sugars, mainly glucose, as they pass through the small intestine. Glucose is then absorbed into the bloodstream, and this glucose-enriched blood flows immediately around the pancreas, stimulating the release of insulin. Even though other factors also contribute to the release of insulin, the rule of thumb is that the more sugar we consume, the greater the amount of insulin is released to help utilize this sugar.

## Glucose in the Body

Utilization of glucose generally means two things: to produce energy to support bodily functions and to store excess glucose for future use. The body is amazingly efficient in this process. It will utilize only what it needs to cover its energy expenditure. Whatever is left over (please recall the law of conservation of energy!) will be stored under the watchful eye of insulin.

Excess glucose can be stored in two ways. First, molecules of glucose can be linked together, forming the glucose-storage depot *glycogen*. Second, when the glycogen stores are fully replete, the remaining molecules of glucose can be converted into fat to be stored in fat tissue. It would be okay to store energy today for tomorrow's use—for a rainy day, so to speak. The problem is, in the land of plenty, this rainy day will never arrive. We continue to consume food and, therefore, energy in excess of our needs on a daily basis. As we consume more and more beyond what we can expend, insulin will gladly do its job—stimulate the storage of more and more glucose and fat in the body. Glucose is stored in the liver and in the muscle, but fat . . . oh boy, don't we know where *that* is stored!

The sixth Draznin Rule is as follows: What doesn't kill makes fat! This is actually an old South African proverb that was conveyed to me by a colleague, an excellent endocrinologist and a native of South Africa, Dr. Mervyn Lifschitz. I have adopted this saying as an important rule.

*The sixth Draznin Rule is as follows: What doesn't kill makes fat!*

Insulin is a life-saving hormone for people with type 1 diabetes, but in everyone else it helps produce fat! Luckily, there is at least one way to minimize the damage. One should, and actually one must, limit the amounts of carbohydrates, especially pure, refined sugars, in the diet. If less sugar reaches the pancreas, less insulin will be released and less energy will be stored as either glycogen or fat.

In contrast to patients with type 1 diabetes who suffer from insulin deficiency, some people with diabetes have enough insulin but it just doesn't work properly. These people require greater amounts of insulin to achieve normal utilization of glucose by their organs and tissues. These individuals are said to have an "insulin resistance." In other words, their ability to utilize glucose as an energy source in response to insulin is reduced. Therefore, they require additional output of insulin to maintain normal levels of sugar in the blood. At some point, these patients fail to produce enough insulin to achieve this goal and they develop type 2 diabetes mellitus (see Table 5.1).

The fact that insulin is needed to ensure normal utilization of glucose is well known to the public. What is much less known, and remains almost unappreciated, is what insulin does in the metabolism of proteins and fats. Without insulin, proteins in muscle break down into individual amino acids, weakening the musculoskeletal system. At the same time,

**Table 5.1  Two Types of Diabetes**

**Type 1**

Usually an autoimmune destruction of pancreatic beta cells with a resultant insulin deficiency. Frequently begins in childhood and in young adults, and insulin treatment is mandatory for survival. Approximately 10% of all patients with diabetes have type 1.

**Type 2**

The cause of this most common form of diabetes is unknown. It frequently begins in adulthood, primarily in individuals who are overweight. It is characterized by inefficient action of insulin (insulin resistance) and inadequate insulin release. Approximately 90% of all patients with diabetes have type 2.

stored fats break down into individual fatty acids and leak out—melting, as it were. A person with a complete lack of insulin rapidly loses weight as a result of the accelerated breakdown of proteins and fats. Without insulin, fat cells will not develop and those cells that have developed previously will lose their fat! In other words, none of us would be able to gain fat mass in the absence of insulin. Conversely, we can only increase our weight if we have sufficient amounts of insulin in our circulation.

Even though insulin is critically important, it is not the only hormone involved in the regulation of weight. Several other hormones and chemical substances in the body help regulate appetite, satiety, and weight maintenance. These include leptin, neuropeptide Y, the melanocortins, ghrelin, and orexins A and B, to name a few. Their presence and their influence also indicate that our expectations of finding a single medicine that will cure obesity in all overweight individuals may not be realistic. There are simply too many factors that influence our ability to gain, lose, and maintain weight. Instead, interventions directed at multiple targets in the complex world of energy balance may be more appropriate and are more likely to be successful.

Signals of satiety and hunger and of thinness and fatness are brought to the brain from the peripheral tissues after being generated in the stomach, liver, gut, pancreas, and fat cells. A very specific area of the brain, a small region known as the "hypothalamus," has been recognized for some time as being responsible for both satiety and eating behavior. In fact, one of the most important hormones, leptin, is produced in fat cells, which collectively constitute one of the largest organs in the body. The word "leptin" comes from the Greek word *leptos,* meaning thin. Leptin is a small peptide that appears to decrease appetite and to increase metabolism. Don't we all wish to have more leptin in the body? Like other peptide hormones, leptin binds to a brain receptor present in the hypothalamus, exerting its influence on the so-called brain satiety center. Leptin's interaction with its receptor signals to the brain that the body has had enough to eat, and as a result, the appetite (the sense of hunger) decreases. In the overall picture, the more fat cells a person has, the more leptin should be produced and the greater the inhibition of appetite should be. In reality, however, it is not always the case. Many obese people have high concentrations of leptin in their bloodstream, but their appetite is not decreased at all. This paradoxical constellation is known as a "resistance" to leptin's action. The causes of this resistance are still unknown.

In the hypothalamus, signals arriving from the body are processed and integrated into various brain centers. The molecules that participate in this process are called "neurotransmitters" as they transmit appropriate information from one brain center to another. One of the most important signals is transmitted by a neurotransmitter known as "serotonin." Experimental evidence suggests that serotonin induces early satiety. Based on this evidence, compounds that stimulate serotonin action have been advocated for the treatment of obesity. For example, a famous (or notorious) combination of phentermine (phen) and fenfluramine (fen) was found to be extremely effective in suppressing appetite; unfortunately, it was also associated with adverse effects that led to its withdrawal from the market.

Overall, it is not unreasonable to foresee that, in ten to twenty years, physicians should have at their disposal medications that will be able to influence appetite, satiety, and eating habits significantly. These new pharmacological agents will, effectively, change both our body weight and our body composition. For the time being, however, the best approach is to embrace the Draznin Rules.

## Turning Food into Energy

Let us now return for a brief moment to the basal metabolic rate (BMR), the amount of energy required to support body functions at rest—when we sleep, for example, or thumb leisurely through the pages of the local newspaper. The more energy we use to support the work of our hearts, lungs, brains and the like (in other words, the higher our BMR), the less energy will remain in our energy stores. As always, the energy we use for the needs of our resting bodies is derived from food. If food is not consumed, either intentionally (for example, during an overnight fast or during an attempt to lose weight) or unintentionally (if one is starving, as a result of either food deprivation or another disease), the energy to provide for the basic functions of the body is mobilized from the energy stores. This energy is initially derived from glycogen (carbohydrates stored in the liver and in muscle), which runs out fairly quickly, and then from fat (stored as fat tissue), which lasts longer.

> *The more energy we use to support the work of our hearts, lungs, brains and the like . . . the less energy will remain in our energy stores.*

Now that we know that the energy to support the life of an organism is derived from foodstuffs, let us briefly review how that actually happens. How does my slice of pecan pie convert into the energy I spend moving from the sofa to the refrigerator?

Dr. Hans Krebs, a scientist who received a Nobel Prize in 1953 for his discoveries of the major steps in the biochemistry of energy production, elegantly divided this process into three stages. Thanks to food labels, everyone now knows that the items we consume are composed of three major nutrients (as we call them, "macronutrients"): proteins, carbohydrates, and fats. In the first stage of energy production from food, large molecules are broken down into smaller units. Proteins are reduced to amino acids; large carbohydrates are converted into simple sugars, such as glucose; and fats are broken down into glycerol and fatty acids. Even though no energy is generated at this point, this is the critical preparatory step as only these simple molecules can be used to generate energy at stages two and three. Certain medications that we use to prevent weight gain or to ameliorate diabetes work specifically at this stage. For example, acarbose interferes with the breakdown of complex carbohydrates into simple sugars, thereby retarding and diminishing the absorption of carbohydrates into the bloodstream.

In the second stage of energy production from food, these smaller molecules enter various cells, and most of them are further reduced or degraded into a very few simple units that enter the *mitochondria*—the energy-making factories of the cells of our bodies. Although some tissues, such as heart tissue, prefer using fatty acids to generate energy, in most cells of the human organism a healthy competition exists between fatty acids and glucose for the privilege of being burnt for the sake of producing new cellular energy.

Stage three is the real factory for production of energy. Remnants of sugars and fats are burnt in the energy-producing furnace to generate energy that is stored in high-energy compounds known as "adenosine triphosphate," abbreviated ATP. The ATP molecules function like a battery, supporting the life of each cell in the body.

Carbohydrates, the most abundant source of calories in the human diet, are present in both plant and animal products, and they are easily broken down into simple sugars for speedy absorption. Carbohydrates are an excellent source of quick energy, with 1 g of carbohydrate providing four calories. Excess carbohydrate is readily stored in the liver and muscles in a form of glycogen that is also easily broken down into single molecules of glucose for quick utilization.

Proteins are built from twenty-two amino acids, eight of which can only be obtained from food. Because these eight amino acids cannot be produced in our bodies, they are termed "essential." The richest source of protein is meat, which, in combination with milk, cheese, and eggs, provides all eight essential amino acids. Many plant foods also contain substantial amounts of protein. Although, like carbohydrates, a gram of protein provides approximately four calories, proteins are rarely used to cover energy needs. They are much more suitable as building materials, to create new proteins in muscle, and everywhere else.

Fat is the most significant metabolic fuel we have. One gram of fat provides nine calories, twice as many as carbohydrates or proteins. Therefore, in terms of acquisition of energy, fat is the most efficient source. It is particularly important for tissues that use great quantities of energy in their work. These tissues are skeletal muscle and heart muscle. For absorption, dietary fats are broken down into single fatty acids and glycerol. In the bloodstream, they travel throughout the body and are either used as a source of energy or deposited in storage, in fat tissue. Approximately 85% of the body's energy is stored as fat.

How is this relevant to what, and how much, we eat? How is it related to our ultimate weight? Or to our ability to lose weight? The answers are complex, but they are directly and critically relevant to the regulation of body weight. According to the law of conservation of energy, if we are to maintain our weight, the energy we generate during these three stages must be equal to the energy we expend. If we generate more energy than we expend, we gain weight. If we expend more energy than we generate, we lose weight. We also have to eat

*If we generate more energy than we expend, we gain weight. If we expend more energy than we generate, we lose weight.*

a well-balanced diet so as to avoid unhealthy competition between the macronutrients. If the diet is not hypocaloric (composed of fewer calories than are expended), the nutrient that is consumed in excess, whether it is fat or carbohydrate, will immediately be placed into storage.

Despite competition, for most body cells it is easiest to use glucose as a source of energy. Glucose is the most readily available source of energy. This simple carbohydrate is critical for providing energy to the brain, the muscles, the liver, the kidneys, and virtually every organ and every cell in the body. As a source of energy, glucose can be utilized immediately to generate energy or placed into storage, as glycogen, a chain of molecules of glucose kept together by chemical bonds. When we fast or exercise, glycogen breaks down, releasing individual molecules of glucose into the energy-production pathway. Unlike plants, animals cannot produce glucose from fat directly. Practically speaking, this means that consumption of a diet with a high fat content cannot raise the blood-sugar levels directly.

In contrast to the production of glucose from fat, the opposite process—the production of fat from glucose—is very much possible in the animal kingdom. After all, bees make fat (wax) from sugar (honey). Piglets grow into large fat pigs and ducklings grow into succulent fat ducks on a carbohydrate-rich diet. This happens because the storage of excess energy in fat is much more efficient than the storage of energy as glycogen (carbohydrates).

In the human, however, this concept has been difficult to prove. Numerous studies have shown only minimal conversion of glucose into fat in human beings. However, in the Central African country of Cameroon, the Guru Walla tribe has an interesting tradition of overfeeding. Guru Walla adolescent boys consume about 7,000 calories in carbohydrates daily, and they gain twelve kilograms (over twenty-six pounds) in ten weeks, while ingesting only a minimal amount of fat.

## Case Study: Mr. G.

Let us now consider the story of Mr. G. Mr. G. is a forty-two-year-old accountant who eats a well-balanced diet, consuming approximately 3,200 calories daily. He does not watch the distribution of fats and carbohydrates in his diet, but he looks for "no cholesterol" items in his favorite grocery store. He leads a fairly sedentary lifestyle, and his walking is limited to the distance from his car to either his office or a grocery store. His BMI is 29, and his caloric expenditure is approximately 2,800 calories per day. He is concerned with a recently accelerated weight gain.

Clearly, as long as his caloric intake (3,200 calories) exceeds his caloric expenditure (2,800 calories), Mr. G. will continue to gain weight. He is said to be in a positive calorie balance (+400 calories), and he will not lose weight, no matter what the composition of his diet is.

At his yearly physical, Mr. G. was found to have cholesterol levels of 290 mg/dl. He began a low-fat diet. He is now buying low-fat yogurt and low-fat cream cheese, he eats pasta twice a day, and he snacks on apples and oranges, consuming about four fruit servings each day. His caloric intake is now down to 2,900 calories. After an initial loss of three pounds, his weight had remained stable for four months; but over the next six months, Mr. G. gained six pounds. His cholesterol came down to 260 mg/dl.

With the best of intentions, Mr. G. replaced calories derived from fat with calories from carbohydrates. His lifestyle did not change, and his diet is still not hypocaloric (low-calorie). Even though he burns carbohydrates, he consumes so many that, in the absence of exercise, the carbohydrate excess is directed to storage and conversion to fat. Mr. G. would derive greater benefit from this new diet if he were to start an exercise program to stimulate his muscles to burn the excess carbo-

*Mr. G. would derive greater benefit from this new diet if he were to start an exercise program to stimulate his muscles to burn the excess carbohydrates.*

hydrates. With Mr. G.'s current lifestyle, a high-carbohydrate diet would lead to a greater weight gain and would not help him with his cholesterol.

Mr. G. has read about an "all you can eat," high-protein, high-fat, low-carbohydrate diet. His coworker lost ten pounds in three weeks on this new wonder diet. Mr. G. eagerly jumped onto the bandwagon. He now eats a three-egg omelet and two servings of meat a day, as well as a lot of cheese, and he drinks a glass of whole milk with each meal. His daily caloric intake is 3,000 calories. After an initial loss of seven pounds over the first month, he maintained his weight for three months and gained nine pounds over the next nine months. He has frequent morning headaches, and he is very tired by the end of the day. His lifestyle has not changed.

Because he stopped consuming carbohydrates, Mr. G. quickly depleted his carbohydrate storage (glycogen) and lost a lot of water that was stored along with the glycogen. This explains his initial weight loss. Mr. G.'s diet is still not hypocaloric. With his glycogen stores depleted, his liver cannot generate sufficient amounts of glucose after an overnight fast. Because glucose, the main energy source for his brain, is now scarce, his liver makes ketones, a chemical product that can be used as a replacement fuel. However, ketones, when produced in excess, can be toxic. With this compensatory *ketosis* (a state of excessive production of ketones), Mr. G. began experiencing morning headaches, and he is becoming excessively tired by the end of the day. In fact, he is so tired that he cannot even think about adding exercise to his daily routine. Mr. G. persists in his mistake of not switching to a hypocaloric diet. Instead, he is currently on a ketogenic diet that worsens his fatigue and introduces a new problem, morning headaches.

## Commonsense Conclusions

What Mr. G. should be doing is quite obvious. He must begin a well-balanced hypocaloric diet and change his sedentary lifestyle. He should consume a daily diet of approximately 2,300 calories, with 40%–45% carbohydrates, 35%–40% fat (mainly monounsaturated and polyunsaturated), and a healthy mix of low-carbohydrate and Mediterranean diets. At the same time, he should start a walking program, building his tolerance to three Draznin Miles a day. This will assure slow but steady and substantial weight loss, an improvement in his lipid profile, and, most important, a lifelong weight-maintenance plan and a healthy lifestyle.

*Chapter Six*

# A Person Does Not Lose Weight by Diet Alone

---

M r. K., whom we met earlier, is sitting in front of me, awaiting recommendations. I see in his eyes that, in his mind, he has already made a commitment to follow my advice. After much trial and error, he wants to give my program a good try. But is Mr. K. a candidate for a low-carbohydrate diet? Would he lose weight, improve his blood-sugar level, and lower his blood pressure? Would he reverse his insulin resistance? Would he reduce his risk of developing heart problems and diabetic complications? Would he stick with the Draznin Mile program, at home and at work, while on business trips and on vacation?

These were the questions that crossed my mind as I listened to Mr. K.'s complaints, carefully examined him, and perused his two-inch-thick medical record—all the while sorting out my approach to his problems. I know what he has to do, but I also know that progress will be difficult for him. To change a lifelong set of habits is not a trivial task.

> *To change a lifelong set of habits is not a trivial task.*

Mr. K. and I are now teammates. We are looking straight into each other's eyes. We have established a common goal: to defeat his obesity and diabetes before they defeat him. With his commitment before us, I make a counter-commitment to him: I will guide him to success. I will be available to him whenever he needs me, and I will use my time and knowledge to lead him to what has now become our common goal.

Every single day, I see patients like Mr. K. in my office. I learned a long time ago that patients without *patience* do not do well. The road to success is filled with frustration and setbacks. I can only promise to do my best to guide them through the roadblocks. They may follow my guidance, but it is up to them to overcome the setbacks. Frustrated people try to diet again and again and again, only to go through the same routine: initial success, followed by a bounce-back after a few short months. No wonder so many individuals give up trying to diet. It is not surprising that people jump on every new gimmick, on every new diet, and on every new pill that purports to help.

National statistics do not lie. They clearly show that almost everyone who starts a weight-loss program loses weight. To lose weight initially has never been a problem. The huge problem is that 90% of dieters regain weight within the first year after an initial weight loss! For many, the yo-yo dieting continues for decades. But I am confident that your efforts will not be in vain if you faithfully embrace the Draznin Rules of lifestyle.

## The Importance of the Hypocaloric Diet

Based on the law of conservation of energy, we can state with confidence that if Mr. K. consumes fewer calories than he expends, he will lose weight. Plain and simple. No miracles. That is why all diets that restrict food intake work. Physicians and nutritionists call these "hypocaloric" diets. *Hypocaloric* means that the diet provides fewer *Hypocaloric means that the diet* calories than are needed to *provides fewer calories than are* cover daily energy require- *needed to cover daily energy* ments. While on these diets, *requirements.* patients consume less energy than they expend. They are said to be "in negative energy balance." In fact, these people have to mobilize additional energy from the storage places—that is, from fat and from glycogen (remember, glycogen is the storage form of sugar)— to meet their energy needs. Spending more than one has leads to a loss, whether in money or in extra pounds of flesh. Hence, we invariably lose weight on hypocaloric diets.

The easiest analogy to help understand the concept of the negative energy balance is your weekly financial balance. Suppose you receive a weekly salary of $500. Even though you have a savings account in your local bank, you are trying to live from check to check, with a weekly budget of $500. Generally speaking, you spend $500 a week for food, housing, car expenses, and other miscellaneous items. If, one week, you have suddenly spent your $500 by Wednesday, the only way you can meet your financial obligations on Thursday and Friday is by withdrawing additional funds from your savings account. You have just found yourself in negative balance. You can exist in negative balance until you deplete your savings account.

Fat around your waist and hips is your energy saving. If you consume less energy than you spend, you will be continuously depleting your fat storage. Unlike the money in the above example, which we wish would grow monthly if not daily, your goal is to deplete your energy savings and get rid of your fat. So the first step in Mr. K.'s new lifestyle program is quite clear: Mr. K. must be put on a hypocaloric diet. But what exactly does that mean?

If you consume precisely the same amount of energy as you spend, you are said to exist on an "isocaloric" diet. In other words, you are in a state of equilibrium, as far as energy is concerned. In this state of equilibrium, you are not going to lose or gain any weight. With the goal of losing weight, what you really wish to know is how much less intake than that of your isocaloric diet you must adopt in order to place yourself in negative caloric balance. The most scientific way to calculate by how much your calorie intake should be restricted is to measure your basal metabolic rate (BMR), and then go on a diet that allows you 300–500 calories less than your BMR.

If we had measured the BMR of Mr. K., we would have learned that it was approximately 2,200 calories. After subtracting 400 calories, I would recommend that he consume a diet of 1,800 calories per day. For him, this number of calories would be hypocaloric. For most people, a diet containing 1,200–1,500 calories is sufficiently hypocaloric, relative to the BMR, and they should lose weight consistently and safely while on such a diet.

Some people begin their dieting with a very low–calorie diet, a diet containing between 400 and 600 calories daily. This is a drastically reduced caloric intake, and one would certainly lose weight like this. However, these diets can be dangerous for people with certain medical problems or even for otherwise healthy individuals. One should consult a doctor before starting such a diet, but even with a physician's blessing, no one should be on one of these very low–calorie diets for longer than ten to fourteen days.

All successful diets are hypocaloric, including every popular diet that you can find on the shelf of your favorite bookstore or on the Internet. Whether you are on the Atkins diet, the Ornish diet, the Zone diet, the South Beach diet, Draznin's dietary principles (after reading this book), or any other diet, you will only lose weight if you consume fewer calories than you expend.

Using a computer program known as the Food Processor SQL nutrition and fitness software, one can easily calculate the caloric content of the popular diets from the menus they recommend. It turns out that the introductory menu of Dr. Atkins contains 1,400 calories per day (including 29 g of saturated fat!) The Zone diet recommends 1,340 calories per day, and the Sugar Busters! diet recommends 1,000 calories per day. Absolutely, undoubtedly, surely, and unequivocally, one will lose weight on any one of these diets! Short-term success is guaranteed.

But if all these diets are hypocaloric, meaning that you eat less, how come some of their advertisements and testimonials tell you that you can eat as much as you want and still lose weight? Do they lie? Not necessarily. But they certainly don't tell you all the truth and nothing but the truth. They play tricks with your appetite. For example, people who are on Dr. Atkins' diet and consume only proteins and fat have livers that will generate a lot of ketone bodies to supply energy to their brains—in order to substitute for the missing glucose usually supplied by carbohydrates.

Ketone bodies suppress appetite. But they can also cause headaches, reduce your ability to concentrate, and make you feel more tired. As a result, you will eat less. With a complete lack of carbohydrates, those who follow the Atkins diet are no longer providing good-quality energy for their brains. Furthermore, a diet completely devoid of carbohydrates can, and frequently does, cause constipation. Fatigue and nausea may be associated with the ketotic state. Many patients on low-carbohydrate diets experience dizziness, and they may have a significant drop in blood pressure when they stand up quickly. A high-protein diet also creates an additional workload for the kidneys, and this could precipitate kidney stones and gout. Beyond that, a diet of only meat and eggs day after day after day doesn't taste that great either. How many strips of bacon and fried eggs can you eat?

Perhaps the biggest problem with the Atkins diet is that we don't really know what kind of damage it can do to our hearts if we manage to stick with it over the long haul. Dr. Atkins honestly believed that no harm would be done by his diet, even if it is consumed for many, many years. In fact, he argued that, in the long run, his diet would reduce blood-cholesterol levels. I believe that Dr. Atkins was only partially correct. His diet may result in lower production of very low–density lipoproteins (VLDLs), which are fats that contain triglycerides and cholesterol. A 50% reduction in VLDL production, for example, will result in an approximately 10% reduction in cholesterol levels. However, unlimited consumption of saturated fat can be extremely detrimental to the heart and blood vessels, even when cholesterol levels are reduced.

*. . . unlimited consumption of saturated fat can be extremely detrimental to the heart and blood vessels, even when cholesterol levels are reduced.*

Overall, until good clinical studies are conducted, it would be prudent to avoid the Atkins diet as a long-term solution.

Dr. Ornish's diet is truly hypocaloric. It eliminates fat and many proteins—essentially all food items with high caloric density. Dieters are advised to eat grains and fibers. But two major problems arise with this diet. First, it just doesn't taste good. After a while, all these wonderful grains, without a trace of fat, become tasteless. No matter how you slice it, this is not an appealing, palatable diet. (At least, not to most of us.) Consequently, it would take an incredible commitment on the part of a patient to adopt the Ornish diet as a long-term solution to his or her needs. The second problem is that if one sticks to this regimen, one is almost constantly hungry. Not only is this diet hypocaloric, but its high carbohydrate content is constantly stimulating the release of insulin. Insulin lowers blood-glucose levels and increases appetite. People on this diet are always hungry and are always munching on granola and other grains that provide only short-term relief. It is both masochistic and heroic to stay on this diet beyond several weeks. The Zone diet is more balanced than either the Atkins diet or the Ornish diet. But it also must be hypocaloric to be successful. While allowing intake of all three major nutrients—protein, fat, and carbohydrate—it limits the overall size of your meal, the size of your meat and fish (no larger than the size of your palm), and the amount of carbohydrates. To stay "in the Zone," so to speak, and not be hungry, you have to consume great quantities of low-caloric fruits and vegetables—in other words, roughage. The Zone diet also has a set of complicated rules that must be followed in order to calculate protein requirements based on several tables and charts. You must also calculate the amount of protein and fat eaten when consuming carbohydrates in order to remain in "the Zone."

## Understanding Dietary Composition

A study that I conducted at the University of Colorado has revealed another interesting finding about the composition of a given diet and its impact on overall dietary effectiveness and ultimate success. We gave our overweight patients a hypocaloric diet—400 calories a day less than was needed to maintain their energy balance in a neutral position. In other words, they had a 400 calorie-a-day deficit compared to what they spent. One half of these patients received a hypocaloric diet low in fat and high in carbohydrate content, while the other half received a hypocaloric diet enriched in fat and low in carbohydrate. Because the diet was hypocaloric, all patients lost weight over a period of sixteen weeks. However, insulin-sensitive patients lost more weight on a high-carbohydrate hypocaloric diet. In contrast, insulin-resistant patients lost considerably more weight on a high-fat hypocaloric diet. This suggests that the state of insulin sensitivity governs individuals' responses not just to diet but also to dietary composition.

Lately, this concept has been supported by a number of studies from other institutions. For example, a group of researchers from Children's Hospital in Boston under the leadership of Dr. David Ludwig demonstrated that a low-carbohydrate diet (40% carbohydrates) was more effective in achieving weight loss in individuals with higher levels of insulin—by definition a group of more insulin-resistant subjects.

After many years of wrangling, and after a meteoric rise and a precipitous fall of the low-carbohydrate fetish, the question of which diet is the best is still an open one. Very recently, Dr. Michael Dansinger and colleagues at the Tufts-New England Medical Center compared head to head the Atkins, Ornish, Weight Watchers, and Zone diets in 160 participants, each randomly assigned to one of these four popular diets. They found that each diet modestly reduced body weight at one year. Not surprisingly, the overall dietary compliance was poor, but better adherence to the diet resulted in greater weight loss. This was true for all four diets, and there was no advantage of one diet over the others.

Somewhat different results were published by a group of clinical scientists from Stanford University. This group, led by

Dr. Christopher Gardner, reported a slight but significantly greater weight loss in overweight and obese women on the Atkins diet than in those on the Zone, Ornish, or LEARN (Lifestyle, Exercise, Attitude, Relationship, and Nutrition—another high-carbohydrate diet) diet at 12 months of follow-up. Longer-term studies are still needed to compare the relative efficacy of these diets.

In summary, the Atkins diet may negatively affect our blood chemistry and hearts, while lifelong converts to the Zone and Ornish diets are hard to find. So if all these popular diets result in weight loss, how come we, as a nation, are becoming more and more obese?

The answer is simple. Nine out of ten dieters, regardless of the regimen they choose, cannot keep up their dietary efforts for long, and certainly not forever. The seventh Draznin Rule is as follows: A person does not lose weight by diet alone. Successful dietary modifications must be accompanied by permanent changes in lifestyle, especially by

*The seventh Draznin Rule is as follows: A person does not lose weight by diet alone.*

exercise. Statistically speaking, the only dieters who are able to maintain their reduced weight are those who incorporate exercise into their lives. After you have lost weight and shed those unwanted pounds, exercise is the key to success in keeping your body from regaining what you had to work so hard to lose. Let me explain why it is so vitally important.

Today, when the tastiest and the most appealing food items contain high levels of both carbohydrates and fat, we overeat without even noticing it. Our energy reservoirs are constantly filled to capacity. The fat we consume is stored inside our bodies as fat, under the skin and wrapping around our organs, such as the heart, liver, kidney, and so forth.

Fat is our long-term reservoir of energy. It takes time to build up fat deposits, and unfortunately, it takes even longer to get rid of excess. In contrast, for its immediate needs, the body uses energy stored as glycogen, a form of stored carbohydrates. Glycogen is very easily and rapidly made from glucose, in the liver and in muscles. This process is called *glycogenesis,* and it is under the tight control of insulin.

After a meal, complex and not so complex carbohydrates are split into individual molecules of glucose in the gut (intestines). These molecules are then absorbed into the bloodstream and trigger the release of insulin. Insulin pushes glucose into cells and tissues, and it stimulates the deposition of the excess glucose as glycogen in the liver and muscles (the liver picks up glucose without the help of insulin).

Thus, our old friend, insulin, helps build up glycogen stores and prevents glycogen breakdown. In contrast, between meals or during exercise, when the levels of insulin are lowest, glycogen is broken down to provide glucose for the brain and other organs. During fasting or exercise, the levels of insulin are low and cannot prevent glycogen breakdown into individual molecules of glucose, which can now be used as a rapidly accessible energy source by all the organs of the body. Hence, glycogen provides energy for the immediate needs of the organism. When glycogen depots (that is how scientists refer to glycogen storage) are depleted but the body still needs energy, then and only then do fat cells begin to release the fat needed to provide the required energy. The glycogen stores can be depleted in two ways. One way is to eat a low-calorie, low-carbohydrate diet so that insulin will not be able to convert glucose into glycogen. Another way to diminish our glycogen stores is to exercise. Exercise requires energy and stimulates the breakdown of glycogen so as to liberate the molecule of glucose that can be now utilized in the energy-production pipeline. In the absence of glycogen, and with a low-carbohydrate diet, the body will start using fat as the energy source, thereby helping maintain the reduced weight.

What is even more important to understand is the opposite process. When the glycogen depots are completely filled and yet one continues to consume carbohydrates, where do these carbohydrates go? With energy production not in demand and the energy stores filled to capacity, the glucose excess is converted to fat.

Knowing how difficult it is to stay on a hypocaloric, low-carbohydrate diet, it is not surprising to realize that, without exercise, we will almost undoubtedly fail any dietary regimen and regain all those dreaded pounds. Study after study has clearly shown that only people who accepted exercise as a new way of life were able to keep their weight down, years after shedding the extra pounds.

## Diet Plus Exercise

For quite a long time, patients with diabetes and their physicians have realized that exercise, in addition to helping us lose weight, lowers blood-sugar levels. This observation was subsequently translated into valuable practical advice which was given to many patients with diabetes: exercise. At the same time, scientists working in the fields of weight regulation and diabetes wished to know the mechanism of the effect of exercise on blood-sugar levels.

Scientists are very curious people. They wish not only to know that action *A* produces effect *B* but also to learn as much as possible about this

*How exercise helps maintain reduced weight and decrease blood-sugar levels is not a trivial question.*

process and to understand what happens at every step along the way from *A* to *B*. How exercise helps maintain reduced weight and decrease blood-sugar levels is not a trivial question. Better understanding of the cellular and biochemical events accompanying exercise might (and probably will) lead to better treatment options in the future.

Some of the very first experiments with exercise revealed that uptake of glucose by muscle cells can be activated by muscle contractions (which is the essence of exercise!) independently of insulin. Even in insulin-resistant patients—those who did not respond well to insulin—exercise effectively stimulated the entry of glucose into cells, thereby reducing the levels of sugar in the blood. So exercise was found to be able to circumvent the inactivity of insulin and promote the entrance of glucose from the bloodstream into various organs and tissues. What proved to be especially important for patients with diabetes was that, in response to exercise training, their bodies became much more sensitive to insulin. In other words, insulin began working much more efficiently in those insulin-resistant patients who became involved in a long-term exercise program.

Clearly, exercised muscle demands more energy than does muscle at rest. Energy for cellular utilization is produced mainly from glucose, either from new glucose molecules that enter the cell or from glucose stored in the cell and liberated from glycogen, a compound that stores glucose. If one exercises long enough, one begins depleting glycogen stores in order to supply glucose for sufficient production of energy.

Freeing up space in the glycogen store is important in at least two ways. First, with a decline in supplies of intracellular glucose, cells begin using fatty acids as an alternative fuel to produce energy. Fatty acids are derived from fat that breaks down to liberate this alternative fuel. Second, when, some time after exercise, a person consumes carbohydrates, newly absorbed glucose can be deposited in now depleted stores and will not be turned away to be converted into fat.

From a practical point of view, exercise is a superb adjunct to both a weight-treatment program and a diabetes-treatment plan. In and of itself, without an appropriate diet, exercise may not be very successful and certainly is not expected to be curative. But along with diet and medications (as needed), it helps in keeping weight down and controlling diabetes.

*. . . exercise is a superb adjunct to both a weight-treatment program and a diabetes-treatment plan.*

The opposite is also true. Without a meaningful exercise program, diet alone usually fails and the treatment of diabetes is not very successful. Finally, please remember that the three Draznin Miles a day will make all the difference!

*Chapter Seven*

# A Tale of Two Brothers

---

D o you remember how many times your parents told you that your brother behaved better, studied harder, and kept his room much cleaner than you did? They repeatedly pointed out that he even liked homemade soup, when all you wanted was a slice of cheese pizza. By the time you enrolled in high school, you knew pretty well that your brother, Tom, was very different from you. He was, and still is, a very smart nerd. He could spend an entire evening thumbing through the *Encyclopedia Britannica* or solving mind-twisters from *Games* magazine. You, however, with your bountiful energy and awfully short attention span, would rather have played ball, ridden your bike, or played video games. Every time your parents compared you to your brother, you screamed back, "I'm not Tom! I'm not my brother! I'm Johnny!"

The truth of the matter is that you were absolutely correct. You were, and you still are, very different from your brother. And both of you are strikingly different from your parents, distinctly different from your sisters, and a world apart from your cousins. In fact, no one would ever contemplate comparing you with your cousin Harry, and your sister would never be confused with your cousin Sarah. Even though we share many genes with, and may physically resemble, other members of our immediate or extended families, we all are individuals. We have our own *individual* characters, mind-sets, culinary habits, and athletic abilities.

*Even though we share many genes with, and may physically resemble, other members of our immediate or extended families, we all are individuals.*

Why, then, do dietitians and doctors and authors of popular diet books offer one and the same prescription for all of us? Let us now suppose that you and I develop the same disease, hypertension (high blood pressure). It turns out that you and I live in the same neighborhood and go to the same doctor, a friendly and knowledgeable family physician. When you and I visit our doctor, we do not expect to be treated in exactly the same way. The doctor is likely to prescribe different medications for us or, at least, different doses of the same medication. We realize that even though we have the same diagnosis, the disease is acting upon two distinct individuals—you and me—causing somewhat different problems and requiring individualized therapy.

Exactly the same principle applies to recommendations with regard to diet and exercise. They simply cannot, and should not, be the same for everyone. The key is to select the most appropriate regimen for a given patient. Not everyone has to avoid egg yolk, and not everyone must be on chromium and manganese. The amounts of carbohydrate in the diet must be adjusted to the degree of physical activity of the individual person, whereas the amounts of protein must be adjusted according to the ability of the kidneys to handle the protein load.

Although the goal of a physician who treats many patients is uniform—to achieve the best possible control of blood pressure and sugar levels and to design the best program for weight maintenance—the means to reach this goal can be as distinct as night and day. The approach and the means ought to be routinely individualized by paying close attention to the patient's state of mind, physical abilities, tastes, habits, and work and leisure schedules, as well as the presence of other medical conditions.

## Two Brothers, Two Treatment Plans

Here is a fairly straightforward example of how different Tom is from his brother, Johnny. Tom is a forty-six-year-old self-employed plumber who gets his job assignments from a general contractor. He is usually out his door at 6:00 AM after drinking a glass of orange juice and on a construction site forty-five minutes later. His first meal is about 10:00 AM, and lunch is at about 1:00 or 1:30 PM. Both meals are usually eaten at the nearest fast-food restaurant. Tom tries to be home before 6:00 PM, and he eats dinner with his family at 6:30 or 7:00 PM.

Tom is five feet nine inches tall and weighs 190 lb. His body mass index (BMI) is 28. His weight has been stable for the past five years. Two years ago he developed diabetes, which is treated with two pills a day. His fasting blood-sugar levels are still moderately elevated, running at about 150–160 mg/dl, except for weekends, when they go up to 200 mg/dl. His cholesterol and triglycerides are also moderately increased.

His brother Johnny is a forty-nine-year-old clerk with the state motor vehicle department. He eats breakfast at home at 7:00 AM, lunch in the cafeteria at noon, and dinner at home at about 6:30 PM. At home, Johnny is as sedentary as his brother, mainly watching TV and thumbing through his favorite magazines. However, unlike Tom, who toils on construction sites five days a week, Johnny is sedentary at work as well, spending eight hours at his desk and occasionally taking a leisurely stroll to the men's room. Johnny is five feet ten inches tall and weighs 215 lb. His BMI is 31. He has had diabetes for five years, and despite therapy, his blood-sugar levels constantly hover near and above 200 mg/dl. His lipids are significantly elevated; his blood pressure is mildly elevated.

### Discussion

Both Tom and Johnny are overweight and have diabetes. Both brothers have elevated lipids and higher than normal blood pressure. Johnny's BMI is in the obesity range, most likely because he leads a much more sedentary life than his younger brother does. Tom is very active during work hours, and his sugar levels are lower because of the vigorous manual labor he is engaged in five days each week. Neither brother pays much attention to his diet. More severe obesity and higher sugar levels are probably responsible for higher lipids and blood pressure in Johnny. What shall we recommend to Tom and Johnny? If we look solely at the diagnoses, the two brothers appear to have the same disease. One may even assume that they should be treated in an identical manner.

This assumption would be incorrect and far from the reality of the situation. Tom should start by bringing lunch from home, instead of eating on the go, gobbling up hamburgers and pizzas. Because he is so active, his daily caloric intake should probably stay at about 3,000 calories. I would encourage him to do three Draznin Miles on Saturdays and Sundays and two Draznin Miles twice a week on weekdays. With just a little more structured exercise and better nutrition, Tom should do very well. Obviously, adjustments will have to be made if Tom's blood sugar and lipids do not drop to normal levels, despite the changes in diet and exercise. He may need to start taking lipid-lowering medications if his cholesterol remains higher than is optimal for patients with diabetes. In addition, Tom should definitely stop drinking beer on weekends.

Johnny, however, has a much longer way to go to reduce his weight and to improve his diabetes, blood pressure, and lipid levels. His diet should be reduced to approximately 2,200–2,500 calories, consisting of no more than 45% carbohydrate, mainly as vegetables, fruit, and fiber. He must also begin an exercise program, building to three Draznin Miles five days a week, as described earlier in this book. He might also benefit from meditation exercises, which could help lower his blood pressure. Johnny should start antihypertensive and lipid-lowering therapies right away. Just like his younger brother, he should forget about drinking beer or other alcoholic beverages.

*. . . despite fairly similar conditions, Tom and Johnny should get individualized therapies even before medications are considered.*

As you can see, despite fairly similar conditions, Tom and Johnny should get individualized therapies even before medications are considered. Their diets may be extremely different, and they should be tailored to their individual tastes and food preferences.

## Getting Individualized Care from Your Doctor

After thirty years of practicing medicine, I have not yet seen two identical patients in my examining room, even though some of my patients have been identical twins! I assure you that the concept of designing treatment based on the individual and his or her life circumstances is not some sort of "holistic medicine" substituted for traditional medicine. Physicians incorporate individual patient adjustments into their practices every single day. It is necessary to consider important elements of a patient's life while formulating a thorough assessment and a treatment plan. The advent of managed care, however, has increased the pressure to provide low-cost health care, and this prevents some primary care physicians from spending any extra time with their patients to discuss these topics. Doctors are pressured to see more patients in the course of their eight- to ten-hour workdays, and they are not reimbursed for discussing modes of exercise and dietary habits with their patients.

A meaningful discussion of lifestyle modifications cannot be accomplished in five or ten or even thirty minutes. The American Diabetes Association (ADA), a premier health-care organization in this country, issues a yearly compilation of its clinical recommendations, designed to serve as guidelines for both patients and their physicians, as far as standards of therapy are concerned. These recommendations indicate that at the time of the initial visit of a patient with diabetes to his or her doctor, the physician must take a comprehensive medical history; perform a meticulous physical examination; collect the details of previous treatment programs, including nutrition, exercise, and self-management education; and obtain information on eating habits, nutritional status, and weight history. At the end of the visit, according to the ADA guidelines, a physician shall formulate both short- and long-term goals, outline medical and nutritional therapies, discuss lifestyle changes as needed, offer an exercise prescription, and review self-management issues.

If your doctor is doing all this, you are in good hands. Stay with him or her. Unfortunately, this may not happen too often

*. . . to receive the highest quality of care, one must often see a specialist — an endocrinologist or a diabetologist.*

in the primary care setting. Even the best primary care doctors frequently do not have time to accomplish all these tasks. Therefore, to receive the highest quality of care, one must often see a specialist—an endocrinologist or a diabetologist.

Recently, intriguing and revealing statistics from the Third National Health and Nutrition Examination Survey (NHANES III) were published by Dr. Maureen Harris, of the National Institutes of Health. A national sample of 733 adults with type 2 diabetes demonstrated that 95% of these patients had primary care providers, 88% had two or more physician visits annually, and 91% had health-care insurance. Moreover, very appropriately, 88% of these patients had been screened for hypertension and 84% for lipid abnormalities. So far, so good, right? Everything about this group of people indicated a high quality of care. However, the outcomes of the care were much less satisfactory. Forty-five percent of these adults were obese, with BMI levels of over 30; 58% had poor control of their diabetes, with $HbA_{1c}$ (glycosylated hemoglobin—this is a measure of glucose control where values over 6.5% are considered abnormal) over 7%; 60% of those with high blood pressure and abnormal lipids were not controlled to accepted levels, and 22% of the patients still smoked cigarettes. To me, these statistics are very telling. They speak loudly to the fact that primary care physicians do not have adequate time to devote to patient education and to the problems of their patients' lifestyles.

Excellent and dedicated physicians in primary care practices are at a terrible disadvantage when it comes to the amount of time they can spend with their patients because the current system of health-care delivery is less than optimal. That is why, in the current health-care environment, your family doctor may not be able to direct you properly through the maze of medicinal and dietary choices and other lifestyle-related decisions. Simply put, he or she has no time to do it.

You, however, as a patient or as a consumer, are hungry for this type of information and guidance. That is why you purchased this book and numerous other diet and health guides. You are swimming all alone in this sea of information, searching for a magic lifeboat that will rescue you from the deadly current of your negative lifestyle.

## Two Patients, One BMI

Before we end this chapter, I would like to acquaint you with two of my patients, Mr. T. and Ms. E. Both were significantly overweight, and they had identical BMI levels of 38. But that was where the similarities ended. Mr. T. was a professor of English literature at the local college, a well-educated man, forty-five years of age, with high blood pressure and gout, and with a long list of psychological problems related to a lack of self-confidence and self-esteem. In contrast, Ms. E. was a twenty-one-year-old single mother of three, with no other health problems, juggling a full-time job in a grocery store with evening classes in a community college, while living under extreme socioeconomic pressure.

The fact that these two patients had identical BMI values had very little to do with the choice of therapy for them. The genetic bases for body size, metabolism, feeding habits, and physical activity—the mechanisms that had caused their obesity, their psychological profiles, their social and economic environment, and their health histories—dictate the selection of therapy.

We are still a long way from complete understanding of how these factors, either individually or in concert, influence weight maintenance and energy balance in a given patient. Sooner or later, you too will discover that there is no magic cure-all. There is only knowledge and your own willpower.

*Chapter Eight*

# Treatment of Obesity

---

Weight loss is really all about weight maintenance. Granted, it is difficult to shed extra pounds, but most people can do it over a short period of time. What proves to be exceptionally challenging, as I've said already earlier in this book, is keeping the new reduced weight and not bouncing back to the prediet existence.

How do we treat obesity? How are we going to advise Mr. K., who is so eager to combat his weight problem? What do we say to thousands of others with similar problems? The very first step in considering a multitude of therapeutic options is to modify our attitudes toward obesity (see Table 8.1). By "our attitudes" I mean the attitudes both of physicians *and* of patients.

Society must accept obesity as a chronic health condition and not just as a manifestation of weakness or sloth. Historically, obese individuals have been considered unmotivated, ugly, and somewhat lazy people who are unable to control their voracious appetites.

> *Society must accept obesity as a chronic health condition and not just as a manifestation of weakness or sloth.*

**Table 8.1 Treatment of Obesity**

| Step 1 | Modify your attitude toward obesity |
|---|---|
| Step 2 | Set realistic goals |
| Step 3 | Assess your mental readiness |
| Step 4 | Find a knowledgeable and willing physician |
| Step 5 | The Draznin Mile |
| Step 6 | The Draznin Calorie |
| Step 7 | Modify your eating habits |

Ironically, this perception is strongly supported by the numerous diet books that create the impression that losing weight is an easy, simple, and trivial task. These books offer recipes for losing weight. Their authors imply that the key to losing weight is widely known—it is in your hands, right in front of your very eyes, jumping out at you from the pages of their best-selling books. The implication is that obese people, those gargantuan monsters, simply lack either interest in losing weight or the willpower to become slim and handsome. Even though the recipe for losing weight is readily available to them, these thankless and thoughtless creatures pass up this wonderful opportunity and simply do not wish to become masters of their own fate.

"I have lost eighty pounds," says a smiling thirty-five-year-old woman from a full-page ad. "You can do it too!"

"I've lost thirty pounds in thirty days!" screams another testimonial. "And I'm *never* hungry!"

Not surprisingly, everyone who believes these statements looks at the obese man or woman with astonishment and with questions. If losing weight is so simple, how come we can't do it?

## Easier Said than Done
The truth of the matter is that it is extremely difficult to lose weight. Obese people and those who treat them know this.

Losing weight and keeping it off isn't simple at all; it is profoundly complex and exceedingly difficult. It should not and cannot be trivialized. The treatment of obesity is one of the most frustrating experiences in all of medicine. In many cases, obesity cannot, and will not, be cured. At the present state of clinical and scientific knowledge, we have no cure for obesity, just as we cannot cure diabetes or hypertension—we can only treat them. We can improve, control, and certainly ameliorate the health problems associated with obesity, but cure it? I seriously doubt it. Not yet, anyway.

I submit to you that when I hear my patients say "Doctor, but I cannot exercise!" or "Doctor, I just cannot be on a diet," I do not dismiss these statements lightly. Not all of us can play the violin. Not all of us can draw pretty pictures. Not all of us can pitch a baseball (without even mentioning speed and strike zone). Why, then, do we expect that all of us should be able to enroll in an exercise class?

Conceivably, because of their genetic makeup, certain individuals "select" to avoid physical activities. Surely, they can be forced to exercise, but of their own volition, they won't. Even if they are fully aware of all the potential benefits of exercise, some people just cannot do it. I would safely bet my nickel that most of us would not continue with violin lessons either. One could argue that this parallel is inappropriate because playing the violin requires talent, while exercising requires only perseverance. Not true. No matter what type of activity you enroll either yourself or your children in, chances are that the majority of the enrollees will drop out within a year, be it a cooking class or a music lesson or a foreign language club.

We tend to select activities that we enjoy, and we are therefore more likely to continue with them. For some of us, exercise or a new, healthier diet could never become an enjoyable part of our lives. It will always be a chore, always a struggle, always a pain. This is precisely the reason for the incredibly high attrition rate from the various diet and exercise programs. In fact, in one nationwide study, when overweight individuals were offered enrollment in a weight-reduction program and were given *free* medications, the attrition rate at the end of a year was a whopping 30%! Thirty percent of people dropped out, despite *free* medications and specialized attention to their health care. Truth *is* stranger than fiction.

## Realistic Expectations

Recalling that the ideal body weight is the weight associated with the least adverse health consequences, we should aspire to achieve this modest goal and not to win the swimsuit competition at the local beach club. So, the second step in our treatment of obesity is to set realistic goals. Most experts agree that losing 5%–15% of initial body weight is both realistic and achievable; other experts in obesity assert that losing just 5%–10% of the initial body weight and keeping it at that level for one full year is a commendable goal. Weight loss of this magnitude also automatically improves many of the health problems associated with being overweight.

*. . . the second step in our treatment of obesity is to set realistic goals.*

For instance, if Ms. Q., who tipped the scale at 200 lb, could lose twenty pounds and maintain herself at 180 lb for a year, she and her doctor should be congratulated. At that point, the new and slimmer Ms. Q. and her physician may set new goals. However, if she expects to shed seventy pounds and go down from 200 to 130 lb—and keep that weight off indefinitely— she will most likely fail, never achieving these unrealistic expectations. We should realize that quick fixes, just like get-rich-quick schemes, have never worked and never will. Both patients and their physicians should be well prepared for a long haul, with lifestyle modifications being the key to their success.

The third step in the treatment of obesity (please note that we haven't used any medications or special diets yet!) is to assess whether a patient is mentally and emotionally ready to initiate serious therapy. This state of readiness for behavioral change is crucial in an overweight person because if a patient is not ready to make a major commitment to weight reduction, none of the programs will work. The weight-loss process requires full concentration and sustained effort, so it should not be initiated when other major problems, such as family or financial matters, are dominant in a person's life. This person will simply fail to devote the necessary effort and commitment to his or her weight problems while encumbered with other important concerns. Not surprisingly, instead of a positive outcome, the patient will face yet another defeat, with the ensuing emotional consequences.

*The third step in the treatment of obesity . . . is to assess whether a patient is mentally and emotionally ready to initiate serious therapy.*

Once a patient makes a commitment to change his or her lifestyle toward defeating obesity, the fourth step is to find a physician who has time to deal with these problems and to guide the patient toward reasonable goals. This is not a trivial task in the era of health-maintenance organizations (HMOs)!

*. . . the fourth step is to find a physician who has time to deal with these problems and to guide the patient toward reasonable goals.*

While people whose body mass index (BMI) levels are under 30 can probably benefit from self-directed diet and exercise programs, those with a BMI between 30 and 40 must seek professional guidance as it is highly unlikely that they will succeed on their own. My experience is that nine out of ten patients in this latter weight category will fail to achieve even minimal success without appropriate guidance. There are too many pounds to be lost and too many skills to be learned and applied correctly. Patients with BMI levels over 40 will most likely benefit from bariatric surgery, a procedure that surgically minimizes the size of the stomach and the amount of food that can be consumed and absorbed.

Self-guided therapy, the weight-loss program that patients can pursue on their own, basically consists of careful attention to diet, eating habits, and exercise. Number one, *numero uno,* the key element, the cornerstone of all and every weight-reduction diet is that the diet must be hypocaloric. If this condition is not met, one might as well kiss all other efforts goodbye. There will be no miracle of weight loss. No one can circumvent, overcome, or alter nature's law of conservation of energy. If a diet is not hypocaloric, there will be no success and no weight loss. So if you see or hear an advertisement for a pill that will help you lose weight while eating anything and everything you wish, don't believe it, even for a second. If you swallow the bait and decide to waste your money to buy this "wonder pill," you will be taken for a ride.

Recently, while I was in line to pay for my groceries, I read an article in one of the popular magazines that attracted my attention. Written by a dietitian, the article informed the reader that if one maintains a diet of 1,400–1,600 calories, no food is forbidden. One can eat anything and still lose weight, as long as one stays within this range of total caloric intake.

Theoretically, this statement might be true, but in a practical sense it is grossly misleading. You simply cannot eat an 800-calorie piece of rich birthday cake in one sitting and maintain a 1,400-calorie diet. You would either eat almost nothing else for the rest of the day and remain hungry until the next or overeat at the next meal (which is exactly what is going to happen!).

The next several steps in treating obesity are all bundled together. They ought to be entertained simultaneously. Each day, one must start eating approximately 500–1,000 calories per day *less* than one expends during that day. Most obese men will lose about a pound a week by consuming around 1,800 calories a day. Most women would lose the same on a 1,400-calorie diet. Losing a pound a week doesn't sound like much, but multiplying this modest loss by the number of successful weeks, one can expect to lose twenty-six pounds in six months, or fifty-two pounds in a year! This is a very substantial weight loss. At the same time, we should realize that it is very difficult to keep to a nutritionally sound diet on less than 1,200 calories per day. The diet of 1,200 calories or less must be fortified with vitamins and minerals, as described below.

Along with a hypocaloric diet, you must embark on an exercise routine and build up to three Draznin Miles a day, as described earlier in the book. The three Draznin Miles must become an integral part of life, like brushing your teeth or washing your hands. That won't happen in a day or in a week or even in a month. But it might happen in a year. That is where true commitment to lifestyle change comes into play.

Another key component of a successful transition to a "leaner life" is the modification of eating habits. In addition to commitment, this one requires education and knowledge of nutrition. Given a choice, most people in the Western world will select food with 40% fat, up to 20% sugar, and variable amounts of high–glycemic index food items (the concept of the "glycemic index" is discussed in more detail in Chapter 11).

You need to know the reason for changing your long-standing eating habits, how to change them, and what will replace the habits that are no longer healthy. You will have to change when, where, and how you eat. You have to be honest with yourself and carefully write down what you eat and when you eat it. Then you will identify what you actu-

*You will have to change when, where, and how you eat. You have to be honest with yourself and carefully write down what you eat and when you eat it. Then you will identify what you actually wish to change and can begin working on it, one thing at a time.*

ally wish to change and can begin working on it, one thing at a time. For example, if you identify that you eat while driving or watching TV, this can be stopped first, before you introduce other modifications. Every week you should have a written plan for your modification goals.

Recently, a telling statement appeared in a review of the influence of dietary composition on energy intake and body weight, written by doctors at Tufts University in Boston: "Although data from comprehensive long-term studies are lacking, published investigations suggest that the previous focus on lowering dietary fat as a means for promoting negative energy balance has led to an underestimation of the potential role of dietary composition in promoting reductions in energy intake and weight loss." In my view, this convoluted admission of the failure of past recommendations is an understatement. Clearly, replacement of dietary fat with great quantities of carbohydrates has played a major role in the epidemics of obesity we encounter today.

One way to understand whether eating behavior is important to the prevalence of obesity is to understand human eating behavior. Most commonly, three aspects of eating behavior have been studied most. These are restraint, disinhibition, and hunger. Dietary *restraint* is defined as a tendency and ability to conscientiously restrict food intake. This is exactly what dieters do: They restrict their food intake either to lose weight or to prevent weight gain. This restraint is voluntary, and it relates either to quantity of food or to the type of food one wishes to restrict. *Disinhibition* is the tendency to overeat palatable food items either simply in the presence of these items or as a result of other disinhibiting stimuli, most commonly emotional distress. Finally, *hunger* is a powerful signal for food intake that can easily override voluntary restraint.

Notwithstanding the importance of the interplay between hunger and restraint, higher disinhibition has been strongly associated with greater weight gain. Because the presence of our favorite dishes before our eyes is one of the most powerful disinhibiting stimuli, it is clearly one of the most important factors in our eating behavior. Everyone is guilty of this—I'm not sure I can restrain myself when a scoop of chocolate ice cream is placed in front of my eyes. The best way to deal with disinhibition is to avoid buying the high–caloric density items we have previously enjoyed so much.

Depression or emotional imbalance can contribute significantly to overeating. Many people lose control of their eating patterns when they are struggling with problems at work or at home or when they slip into depression.

## The Energy Value of Foods

At the same time, you should learn about the energy values of different food items. You should understand how to evaluate nutrition labels so as to determine the caloric content of the food you consume. Food labels are not as simple as they appear at first glance. They give you the amounts of nutrients in grams in one serving, the serving size, and those nutrients' percentage of a daily 2,000-calorie diet. For example, the label of an item you are considering buying tells you that a single serving contains 12 g of fat and that that represents 18% of the recommended daily value.

You must understand that if you were to eat a 2,000-calorie diet, you could consume 65 g of fat a day. If you ate this particular item with its 12 g of fat for breakfast, you would have the rest of the day at your disposal to eat the remaining 53 g of allowed fat (65 g − 12 g = 53 g). Sixty-five grams of fat will provide you with 585 calories (65 g × 9 calories/g = 585 calories), which will represent 30% of the 2,000-calorie diet. Even if you memorize grams and percentages for a 2,000-calorie diet, it would be difficult to calculate precisely what you have to eat. And then, if you are placed on a 1,500-calorie diet, all the calculations would have to be done anew.

Here is a practical example of how you actually do it. Ms. J. was placed on a 1,500-calorie diet, with the following composition of nutrients: carbohydrates 45%, fat 35%, protein 20%. This meant that she should receive 675 calories from carbohydrates (1,500 calories × 45% = 675 calories), 525 calories from fat (1,500 calories × 35% = 525 calories), and 300 calories from proteins (1,500 calories × 20% = 300 calories).

Now we have to recall that 1 g of fat yields nine calories, whereas 1 g of carbohydrates and proteins each yields four calories. Upon dividing 675 calories by 4, Ms. J. will discover that she can eat 168 g of carbohydrates daily. In a similar manner, she will calculate that she can eat 58 g of fat and 75 g of protein.

Armed with this information, Ms. J. decides to eat for breakfast one serving of food that contains 25 g of carbohydrates, 15 g of fat, and 20 g of protein. She knows that this meal (breakfast) will supply her with 315 calories. She now also knows that during the rest of the day she may still eat 143 g of carbohydrates, 43 g of fat, and 55 g of protein. She can now plan very carefully what she will eat for lunch, dinner, and snacks. But, most of all, she realizes that she can follow this diet only if she plans it in advance.

Is that difficult? You tell me. I think it is. At least, it is by no means easy. Can one do it? Can you do it? The answer is yes, one can, and you can. You don't have to be a rocket scientist, but this is where your commitment and perseverance really count. You will have to write down everything that enters your mouth. You will have to calculate the amounts of macronutrients and the number of calories in every serving you put on your plate. You will have to do that, at least initially, in order to learn what to eat and how much to eat. This learning curve is absolutely critical for your ultimate success.

If you were one of my patients, I would meet with you weekly, or even more often, until your dietary regimen became crystal clear to you. We would go over your dietary recall (a list of the items you eat) and your calculations to ensure you were eating the desired number of calories composed of the desired amounts of carbohydrates, proteins, and fats. Since you are reading this book and so are probably not one of my patients, can you count on the help of a primary care physician? I certainly hope you can, but I wouldn't bet on that. There is nothing wrong with your primary care physicians. I am convinced they are excellent doctors. Unfortunately, as I mentioned before, primary care physicians simply do not have time in their busy daily schedules to devote even ten minutes to these calculations. They refer their patients to dietitians, who know nutrition and who are excellent in their field, but they do not know your specific disease. The vicious cycle begins again—patients are left to fend for themselves, perusing the diet books and self-improvement magazines.

## Medications and Other Chemicals

What about diet pills? Do we have a magic bullet that can kill our appetites, melt our fat, and boost our energy expenditure? That would be ideal, wouldn't it? The reality, however, is that such a pill is a long way away. Today, we have nothing like that. Not yet. Such a miracle treatment is still a dream for many patients and for scores of drug companies that would love to offer such a panacea to a "hungry" public.

Currently, only two drugs, Meridia (sibutramine) and Xenical (orlistat), are approved by the Food and Drug Administration (FDA) as long-term therapeutic agents for obesity. Sibutramine works by blocking the absorption by nerve cells of certain chemicals in the brain, which has been shown to result in inhibition of food intake in experimental animals and in humans. In one well-designed study, patients who took sibutramine lost 8% of their initial weight compared with a loss of only 1%–2% in patients who received a placebo (a sugar pill with no active ingredient). Most important, the weight loss was still present after twelve months of therapy.

*Currently, only two drugs . . . are approved by the Food and Drug Administration (FDA) as long-term therapeutic agents for obesity.*

Side effects of sibutramine are usually mild and disappear rapidly, after the drug is discontinued. The most common side effects include dry mouth, headache, constipation, and poor sleep. In many patients, however, physicians have also observed increased heart rate and a mild increase in blood pressure. For these reasons, blood pressure and pulse must be carefully monitored in patients taking sibutramine. Not surprisingly, as a result, sibutramine should not be given to patients with poorly controlled hypertension, irregular heartbeat, or certain other heart conditions. It should also be used with great caution in patients with glaucoma, in patients with migraine headaches, and in those being treated for depression.

Another way to treat obesity with medications is to attempt to block absorption of fats from the gastrointestinal tract. The idea is that one can eat fatty food and, at the same time, take a pill that will prevent absorption of these fats from the gut (intestines) into the bloodstream. The fat will stay in the gut and will eventually slide down through the loops of the intestine and be evacuated. Xenical (orlistat) is such a drug. It works by blocking absorption of fat from the gut by as much as 30%. In clinical studies, orlistat produced an average loss of 10% of the initial weight, and it was very effective in weight-maintenance programs for up to two years with continued use of the medication.

One caveat is that patients taking orlistat should limit the amount of fat in their diets to less than 30%. Otherwise, large amounts of unabsorbed fat will cause oily stools. With so much fat, the stool will slide down the intestine, reaching your undergarment faster than you can reach the nearest toilet! These patients will have an urge to relieve themselves very frequently (this is called "fecal urgency"), and to their great displeasure, they will not always be able to hold it in ("fecal incontinence"). This is a very unpleasant, embarrassing, and annoying side effect, indeed! Limiting the fat content of the diet will help prevent this side effect.

You probably remember that, several years ago, "fen-phen" was a promising combination of two medications (fenfluramine and phentermine) that suppressed appetite. This medical regimen became extremely popular among both physicians and diet-conscious patients. The drugs, however, were found to cause infrequent but severe side effects (such as heart valve problems) and were pulled off the market.

Lately, a great deal of interest has been shown in the potential effectiveness of herbal medications—in particular, a "natural fen-phen" or "herbal fen-phen" has become exceptionally popular. The term "natural" or "herbal" fen-phen refers to a combination of Saint-John's-wort and ma huang, an ephedra herb. When used separately, the former is generally praised for its antidepressant properties, whereas the latter is a mild to moderate stimulant. Together, they are reported to be helpful in curbing appetite. No scientific evidence, however, exists to support this claim. Incidentally, herbal remedies are not without hazard. Lately, ephedra has been under scrutiny for possibly contributing to the death of several prominent athletes who exercised strenuously in the heat of summer while taking this substance.

For those of you who are eager to use prescription and over-the-counter medications to fight your weight problems, it's important to keep in mind that the long-term safety of these medications is in most cases completely unknown. Furthermore, how long does a medication (even the most benign one) need to be taken? Will three months suffice? A couple

*For those of you who are eager to use prescription and over-the-counter medications to fight your weight problems, it's important to keep in mind that the long-term safety of these medications is in most cases completely unknown.*

of years? Perhaps twenty years? Will the long-term use of these medications improve or impair health? We simply do not know.

Finally, one should realize that patients with a BMI greater than 40 who have failed to lose weight with various behavioral and pharmacological approaches should consider surgery as a viable option in treating their obesity. The number of weight-reducing surgeries (they are known as "bariatric surgeries") is increasing rapidly (by up to 40% each year) as more and more people consider this option. In 2004, 120,000 bariatric surgeries were performed in the United States, while in 2006 the number of bariatric surgeries exceeded 200,000.

Today, two types of surgery are usually performed in obese individuals: gastric restriction and gastric bypass. *Gastric restriction* is a procedure that creates a small pouch in the stomach that basically restricts the amount of food the stomach can receive, thereby limiting one's caloric intake. Smaller amounts of digested food continue to move along the normal route of the remainder of the gastrointestinal tract. In the *gastric bypass* operation, the major part of the stomach and the small intestine are surgically bypassed, thus also reducing absorption of nutrients.

Both procedures, regarded realistically, result in approximately 40% weight loss, with good long-term maintenance. Weight loss in these patients is associated with significant improvement in diabetes, hypertension, breathing disorders, and mobility. The latest analysis of published outcomes suggested that a special type of gastric bypass, called "Roux-en-Y," reversed diabetes in 84% of obese diabetic patients who underwent the procedure. Surgery, however, is not without complications, and one should select a medical center and physician specializing in this type of surgery. It goes without saying that surgical candidates must be fully informed of potential complications. Many centers require that patients go through a thorough psychiatric evaluation to estimate their strength of commitment and ability to cope.

## Medicating Prediabetes

As the old concept of prediabetes reemerged in clinical medicine and the scientific literature, many physicians and their patients began pondering an important question: Should prediabetes be treated with medications in order to prevent its transition to full-blown diabetes? Lifestyle changes prevent the development of diabetes in 50%–70% of patients with prediabetes. Will medications do the same? Will they be equally effective? And if so, what medication should we use? Will there be side effects of these medications in the long run?

Because many patients with prediabetes are either unwilling or, for whatever reason, unable to modify their lifestyle, the search for a "magic pill" continues in the laboratories of almost all pharmaceutical companies. It is easier for a busy doctor to prescribe a pill than to get involved in a long, tedious, and frequently frustrating effort to modify a patient's lifestyle. Unfortunately, today only one drug available on the market offers some reasonable benefit in preventing diabetes. This medication is metformin, and it is also used to treat diabetes. Metformin is currently given to overweight children and adolescents as well as to prediabetic adults. The success of metformin is variable but is somewhere around 35%.

Other medications, such as Avandia (rosiglitazone) or Actos (pioglitazone), may be equally effective; but their long-term safety is not yet established, and their potential side effects do not allow doctors to use them widely. Intuitively, based on common sense and today's scientific information, I would recommend these medications only as a short-term measure, designed to help my patients change their eating habits and their lifestyles. While waiting for a breakthrough in the search for such medications, lifestyle changes and the Draznin Plan remain the best approach to the treatment of prediabetes.

*Chapter Nine*

# What Shall I Do When I Stop Losing Weight Despite My Best Efforts to Keep My Diet and Exercise?

M s. S. is a tall and overweight woman of 38 years of age. She is five feet eleven inches tall and weighs 237 lb. She has been gaining weight steadily from the time of her first pregnancy ten years ago. At some point in the not so distant past, she weighed 267 lb, but with a strict diet and exercise regimen, she lost thirty pounds over approximately eight months. Initially, her weight loss was rapid and visible, improving her mood and motivating her to stay with her new healthy diet and exercise program. She lost twelve pounds in the first month, eight pounds during the second one, five pounds in the third, three pounds in the fourth, and one pound during the fifth and the sixth months each but nothing since. She remains exceptionally strict with her diet and walks almost two hours every day. She has been doing everything she was supposed to do. Not surprisingly, her stalled progress became a source of frustration and disappointment.

What happened? Why did Ms. S. gradually stop losing weight while still adhering to the same regimen that was so successful initially?

These questions are very common, as is Ms. S.'s predicament, among thousands of dieters trying to lose weight. Unfortunately,

98

in the great majority of people, frustration overwhelms their ability to cope and, against their best judgment, they slip off the wagon and return to overeating and underexercising, thus regaining the weight they worked so hard to lose. A slow pace of weight loss or an apparent lack of weight loss after initial success, and the resultant inability of patients to stay with a given program, can be similarly frustrating to a physician.

Some "experts" would nonchalantly say "Eat less and exercise more—that's all there is to it."

Easier said than done. In fact, at this point, when a person has already lost a substantial amount of weight, it is almost impossible to do. As a result, this cavalier advice

*. . . in the long run, the goal of losing weight must become the goal of maintaining the new and reduced weight.*

sounds like a mockery, a mental torture of sorts. This is precisely why, in the long run, the goal of *losing* weight must become the goal of *maintaining* the new and reduced weight.

From a scientist's point of view, it would be both interesting and imperative to understand why and how this new equilibrium develops. Why, after the initial weight loss, do we reach a plateau that seems unresponsive to previously successful measures? If we understand the mechanism, we will be much better equipped to design appropriate therapy, to come up with a plan to reinstill both hope and enthusiasm. For now, however, there is only one way to deal with this problem constructively. It takes time, resolve, and a lot of patience.

## Keeping Goals Reasonable

I tell my patients "Let's lose 5%–10% of the initial body weight and keep the new and reduced weight for at least six months to a year. This initial weight loss is likely to occur within the first six months. Let's not worry for now and not expect to lose a quarter or a third of your weight. Let's lose 5%–10% of your weight and *keep* this loss for six months to a year and consider this a success. The maintenance phase, or period of time during which we want to keep the reduced weight, will then last for an additional six to twelve months. If we are successful in maintaining the initial weight loss over the next six to twelve months, we will then devise a new strategy for an additional 5%–10% weight reduction for the next six to twelve months." With these expectations—that appear modest upon first glance—people are likely to build the necessary confidence, patience, and stamina to acquire a new lifestyle. This is the Draznin Plan at work.

Why it is so difficult to maintain reduced weight is not known, but many researchers in the field of obesity and nutrition are trying to answer this important question. One theory was put forth by two obesity researchers from the University of Colorado, Holly Wyatt and James Hill. They postulated that our bodies have genetically defined requirements for energy expenditure. In other words, the body of a given individual strives to spend a certain number of calories to maintain the work of all organs in the body both at rest (BMR, or basal metabolic rate) and in activity (AT, or activity thermogenesis). As we already know from Chapter 3, the largest share of daily energy expenditure, approximately 50%–65%, is spent on BMR to support the function of brain, muscle, bones, fat, heart, liver, and all other organs in a body. The larger the body is, the greater amount of energy is expended to maintain its functions. Drs. Wyatt and Hill named this difference between the two levels of energy expenditure, pre- and post- weight loss, the "energy gap." They concluded that filling the energy gap with exercise would prevent weight gain and allow the patient to maintain a reduced weight.

Let us consider an example. Mr. X. weighs 200 lb and his energy expenditure is 2,500 kcal a day. He is a sedentary man who is almost never physically active. After a year of dieting, he lost twenty pounds and now weighs 180 lb. Because his body mass is now smaller than it was by twenty pounds, his energy expenditure also went down—let's say to 2,300 kcal. However, according to Wyatt and Hill's hypothesis, his body, now packaged in a smaller frame, retains its genetically predetermined need to spend 2,500 kcal. He can comply with this demand in one of two ways. He can either exercise to burn (expend) an extra 200 kcal and then his total daily energy expenditure will meet the required 2,500 kcal (2,300 kcal plus 200 kcal burned by exercise). Alternatively, he can regain weight back to 200 lb and then his body would burn the required 2,500 kcal without exercising. The price for this second option is heavy—a regain of the initially lost weight.

If Wyatt and Hill are correct and if the "desire" of the body to spend energy is genetically determined and remains relatively constant during a lifetime, then we have no other option but to be sufficiently physically active (to fill this "gap" with exercise) for the rest of our lives in order to maintain a reduced weight. New studies and experiments with cohorts of overweight people are needed to determine whether filling the "energy gap" with exercise is the only option for patients struggling with excess weight. For now, however, *For now . . . a reduction in caloric intake combined with three Draznin Miles each day remains the best recipe for a healthy lifestyle change.* a reduction in caloric intake combined with three Draznin Miles each day remains the best recipe for a healthy lifestyle change.

## Changes in Cognitive Function

Obesity and diabetes are chronic illnesses. Very frequently, chronic illnesses including obesity and diabetes are accompanied by slight changes in cognitive function—so slight that they may be imperceptible to patients and their families. This is particularly true for older people, those over the tender age of 65, and certain elements of cognitive impairment have been observed in 15%–50% of older adults with chronic illness.

"Cognitive function" is a very broad term that encompasses all kinds of thinking abilities, including information processing, the application of knowledge to practical situations, and changing preferences and desires. In many instances, the changes in cognitive function that accompany chronic illness are so subtle that overall mental abilities to work and carry out activities of daily living do not appear to be altered at all. However, imperceptible changes in learning may be serious enough to interfere with or even prevent a person's ability to adapt to a new lifestyle. As a result, even if we health professionals put our best efforts into patient education and patients do their best to learn what they are supposed to do, this newly acquired knowledge often fails to change patients' behavior.

Just as outstanding knowledge of music theory does not equal the ability to play a musical instrument, learning everything about diet, exercise, and diabetes does not equal the ability to effectively combat obesity and diabetes.

The process of acquisition of knowledge is known as "declarative learning." But new knowledge acquired in the process of declarative learning does not directly affect habits. A child can easily learn that one must brush his or her teeth twice a day, but this does not mean the child is going to do it. The acquisition of knowledge is not the same as the acquisition of a habit. A different type of learning, "procedural learning" or "habit-forming learning," is desperately needed to ensure that new knowledge leads to a new lifestyle.

This frequently observed dissociation between acquisition of knowledge about obesity and diabetes and the development of new habits to fight these chronic diseases with a healthy lifestyle may be the result of a mild impairment of cognitive function in these patients.

Another important change in cognitive function frequently seen in patients with chronic illnesses is related to what is known in the world of psychology as "executive cognitive function." The abilities to plan, anticipate consequences of action, initiate purposeful changes and activities, monitor self-action, and detect errors all fall into the category of executive cognitive function. So a person with impaired executive functioning may have difficulties with initiating purposeful changes (such as starting a new lifestyle), inhibiting irrelevant behavior (the habits of the old lifestyle), and monitoring the accuracy of his or her performance. These are all critical elements for self-management of diabetes and for maintaining a healthy lifestyle.

Finally, behavior change requires substantial effort, but effort is difficult. As we all know, it is much easier to do what is habitual. Changing rooted habits in order to defeat obesity and diabetes is exceptionally difficult. Yet building new habits is absolutely critical for the successful alteration of a lifestyle.

*Chapter Ten*

# The Draznin Calorie: A Better Way to Diet

---

Now that we are fully armed with the concept of the Draznin Mile, knowing and accepting that one must log three Draznin Miles a day, we ought to face the second side of the energy-balance equation: the consumption side. What is the maximum caloric intake we can allow ourselves and still lose weight? What would be a sensible dietary limit that assures weight loss initially and weight maintenance afterward? And, most important, how can we practically implement such a program over a long period of time, both at home and while visiting friends or eating out?

The answer to all these important questions is the Draznin Calorie. A *calorie* is scientifically defined as the amount of energy needed to raise the temperature of 1 g of water from 15°C to 16°C (or from 59°F to 61°F). One kilocalorie (or 1 kcal) equals 1,000 calories. The caloric content of food is presented in kilocalories, so the calories we count in our dietary ration are really thousands of those little units of energy needed to heat a gram of water by one degree. For example, 500 calories consumed or expended are 500,000 calories or 500 kcal in "true scientific count."

## A Calorie by Any Other Name . . .

The concept of the Draznin Calorie is quite different from that of both the chemical calorie and the dietary calorie, but it is as simple as the concept of the Draznin Mile. Though this concept is not difficult to understand, it can be incredibly difficult to follow.

Every time the body has an energy deficit (that is, when we expend more energy than we consume), the brain is bombarded with signals of hunger, prompting the body to increase energy intake—in other words, to eat more. The mind and body work in tandem to maintain the energy balance and, if possible, to store extra energy for a rainy day. Therefore, the critical question for every dieter is how to comply with a hypocaloric diet, or even with a balanced diet, in order to lose weight or to prevent weight gain.

The first step of my approach is quite obvious. We must eliminate from the diet all items with high caloric density. These are the items that contain a lot of calories per small amount of food—per bite or per gulp, if you wish. These food items contain large quantities of fat or sugar, such as deep-fried food or nondiet soft drinks and juices. These should be eliminated at once.

After eliminating high-fat and high-carbohydrate items from the diet, the remaining food items can be classified as containing between one and six Draznin Calories per serving. How? Simply look at food labels. They always tell you how many calories per serving the food item contains. Armed with this information, designate any food item that contains fewer than 100 calories per serving as containing one Draznin Calorie. For example, one egg, one

*. . . designate any food item that contains fewer than 100 calories per serving as containing one Draznin Calorie.*

small to medium-sized apple, one slice of whole wheat toast, and one glass of skim milk each contain one Draznin Calorie, regardless of the actual calories present. Sound familiar? (Remember my exercise plan: When you walk for twenty minutes, you cover one Draznin Mile, regardless of the true distance traveled.)

All food items containing between 101 and 200 calories per serving are said to equal two Draznin Calories. Examples include three ounces of poultry or lean meat or fish, one dinner roll, or one cup of lean meat–based soup. Table 10.1 demonstrates the Draznin-Calorie equivalent of the caloric content of certain foods. The eighteen different food items used most commonly by patients adhering to my program are listed in Table 10.2.

The key element of my program is to eat no more than six Draznin Calories per meal and no more than eighteen Draznin Calories per day. Because one Draznin Calorie equals or is less than 100 calories, consuming six Draznin Calories per meal means that one consumes no more than 600 calories. Consuming eighteen Draznin Calories a day assures that the caloric intake for that day will stay below 1,800 calories. Together with walking three Draznin Miles a day, this is an excellent and

**Table 10.1 Caloric Content of Food and Draznin Calorie Equivalent**

| Caloric Content | Draznin Calories |
| --- | --- |
| Up to 100 calories/serving | 1 |
| 101–200 calories/serving | 2 |
| 201–300 calories/serving | 3 |
| 301–400 calories/serving | 4 |
| 401–500 calories/serving | 5 |
| 501–600 calories/serving | 6 |

**Table 10.2 Common Food Items and Draznin Calorie Equivalents**

| Food Item | Draznin Calories |
|---|---|
| 1 egg | 1 |
| 2 breakfast turkey links | 1 |
| 1 slice whole wheat or rye toast | 1 |
| 1 glass skim milk | 1 |
| 3 oz lean meat/poultry/fish | 1 |
| 1 cup vegetables | 1 |
| 1 cup fruit | 1 |
| 1 dinner roll | 2 |
| 1 tsp salad dressing or oil | 1 |
| 1 cup vegetable soup | 1 |
| 1 cup meat-based soup | 2 |
| 1 cup creamy soup | 3 |
| Appetizer (restaurant) | 3 |
| Salad (restaurant) | 2 |
| Entrée-size salad (restaurant) | 4 |
| Entrée without garnish | 3 |
| Entrée with garnish | 5 |
| Dessert | 6 |

efficient way to lose weight. (By the way, if you ate only four Draznin Calories at breakfast, you cannot add the remaining two to your lunch or dinner. Remember that each meal must be no larger than six Draznin Calories. If you eat less, good for you!) Table 10.3 provides an example of a breakfast containing fewer than six Draznin Calories.

The new lean lifestyle is based on spending energy while doing at least three Draznin Miles a day and consuming no more than eighteen Draznin Calories (no more than 1,800 calories). Many of my patients carry a small pocket calendar–sized card with the caloric content of allowable food items in Draznin Calories. Simply by checking off the number of Draznin Calories per meal, they can easily stay within eighteen

**Table 10.3 Sample Draznin Breakfast**

| Sample Breakfast Item | Draznin Calories |
| --- | --- |
| 1 egg | 1 |
| 2 slices toast | 2 |
| 1 turkey link | 1 |
| 1 glass skim milk | 1 |
| Total Draznin Calories | 5 |

Draznin Calories a day and successfully continue with the program.

Restaurant items are typically more caloric than homemade food. Usually, an appetizer in a restaurant contains 300–400 calories, equal to four Draznin Calories. A large entrée-sized salad easily contains 400–500 calories, and this should be counted as four Draznin Calories. A meat, poultry, or fish entrée, usually larger than three ounces, prepared with oils and sauces and served with garnish, equals five Draznin Calories. Desserts cover the entire meal—six Draznin Calories. Based on this count, when eating out, we have several choices (see Table 10.4).

Dinner at home may contain a plate of salad (one Draznin Calorie) with a teaspoon of no-fat dressing (one Draznin Calorie), a dinner roll (two Draznin Calories) and six ounces of grilled chicken (two Draznin Calories), for a total of six Draznin Calories. One can skip the roll and, instead, have either a larger portion of meat or a side dish of vegetables, still staying within the allowable six Draznin Calories.

With this concept of the Draznin Calorie, the only information you need from the food label is the size of a serving and the number of calories per serving. If the number of calories per

**Table 10.4 Sample Dinner Menus**

| Menus | Draznin Calories |
|---|---|
| **Choice 1** | |
| Vegetable soup | 1 |
| Dinner salad | 2 |
| Entrée without garnish | 3 |
| Total Draznin Calories | 6 |
| **Choice 2** | |
| Vegetable soup | 1 |
| Appetizer | 3 |
| 1 dinner roll | 2 |
| Total Draznin Calories | 6 |
| **Choice 3** | |
| Meat-based soup | 2 |
| Large entrée salad | 4 |
| Total Draznin Calories | 6 |
| **Choice 4** | |
| Dessert | 6 |
| Total Draznin Calories | 6 |
| **Choice 5** | |
| Any combination that does not exceed 6 Draznin Calories | |

serving is under 100, simply count it as one Draznin Calorie. If you decide to eat two servings of this food item, you will consume two Draznin Calories. Make a note on your chart, and make sure you eat no more than six Draznin Calories per meal and no more than eighteen Draznin Calories per day. I recommend that you keep an accurate record, in Draznin Calories, of what you eat at each meal; do this for three to four months. During this time, you will develop a habit of eating foods with lower caloric density and in smaller portions. Coupled with a walk of three Draznin Miles a day, you will have developed, and will have learned to maintain, a healthy lifestyle, a slimmer body, and a happier spirit.

Having been so adamant about an individualized approach to my patients' problems throughout this book, I would like to lead you to my practical advice that can serve as the background for your own lifestyle changes. You, or better yet you and your doctor or nutritionist, will be able to modify it, adjusting it to your taste, work and eating schedules, family situation, and other health problems you might have. The diet might appear somewhat stringent, but it isn't. There is a great variety of vegetables and grilled fish and meat to satisfy every hue of every taste. Finally, only two requirements stay constant if one wishes to lose weight: (*1*) one must consume less energy than one expends and (*2*) three Draznin Miles must complement one's dietary efforts.

Now, here it comes—my practical advice.

## Chapter Eleven

# Practical Advice

---

What about alcohol? What about eating out? What foods should you buy, and how should you prepare meals? What about having a dinner at a friend's house? Do you have to take extra vitamins and/or nutritional supplements? Are there, or will there be, any effects on your prescription and over-the-counter medications? All these are important questions. You must know the answers. Fortunately, the answers are simple and reasonable, and the advice is easy to follow.

## Portion Size

Throughout this book I continuously emphasize the importance of a hypocaloric diet as the cornerstone of any lifestyle-changing regimen. As we've already seen, one way to consume fewer calories is to select food items that are lower in caloric content. Another and, in practical terms, perhaps even more important way is to minimize portion size. Avoid eating three large meals a day. In fact, avoid eating large portions, period. If you eat prepackaged food, pay careful attention to a serving size—don't

*Avoid eating three large meals a day. In fact, avoid eating large portions, period.*

eat two servings, always be happy with one. Make your dinner the last meal of the day—do not snack after dinner. Make sure there is always a twelve-hour interval between the last bite of your dinner and the first bite of your breakfast. If you finish your dinner at 9:00 PM, do not eat your breakfast until 9:00 AM. This is a much needed break for your digestion system and a wonderful way to support your hypocaloric diet.

## Added Sugars

The term "sugar" is used to designate both *monosaccharides* (sugars composed of a single molecule) and *disaccharides* (sugars composed of two molecules). The monosaccharides are glucose, galactose, and fructose. The disaccharides include sucrose, lactose, and maltose. Monosaccharides and disaccharides are also known as "simple sugars" or "simple carbohydrates," as opposed to "complex carbohydrates," which consist of many simple saccharide molecules. Many commonly used sweeteners, such as corn syrup, contain trisaccharides, or even longer molecules of saccharides. Complex carbohydrates must be broken down in the digestive tract before they are absorbed into the bloodstream.

*Dietary Guidelines for Americans,* published jointly by the U.S. Department of Agriculture and the Department of Health and Human Services, offers a distinction between "added sugars" and the carbohydrates that naturally exist in food. However, the body cannot make this distinction and treats all sugars, either added or naturally occurring, in the same way. But it is important to understand the term "added sugars" and the impact these sugars have on nutrition. *Added sugars* are defined as sugars that are eaten separately or "added" as an ingredient to processed or prepared food items such as soft drinks, ice cream, cakes, and pies. Added sugars include white and brown sugars, maple syrup, corn syrup, honey, molasses, and fructose sweeteners, to name a few.

Consumption of added sugars in the United States has increased steadily, from 27 teaspoons per person per day in 1970 to 32 teaspoons per person per day at the present time, an increase of 23%. Nine specific food items lead the way in added sugars in the American diet: soft drinks (33%), fruit drinks (10%), candy (5%), cakes (5%), ice cream (4%), ready-to-eat cereals (4%), sugar and honey (4%), cookies and brownies (4%), and syrups and toppings (4%). Soft drinks are the clear winner. Added sugars must be completely eliminated from the diet of anyone who wishes to lose weight.

## Glycemic Index

In 1981, a group of investigators led by Dr. David Jenkins proposed the use of the *glycemic index* (GI) of individual food items in designing an appropriate diet to treat diabetes. The idea was to classify carbohydrate-containing foods numerically, assuming that this might be helpful in treating patients with type 1 diabetes. The concept is fairly simple: Each carbohydrate-containing food item causes a rise in blood-sugar levels, and the magnitude of this rise, relative to the rise elicited by a pure glucose, is the GI of this particular food item. Initial studies by Dr. Jenkins compared changes in blood-sugar levels caused by 50-g portions of various carbohydrates with those caused by 50 g of glucose. The higher the rise in blood-sugar levels after eating a particular carbohydrate, the higher the GI of that carbohydrate.

*The higher the rise in blood-sugar levels after eating a particular carbohydrate, the higher the GI of that carbohydrate.*

Later, a 50-g portion of white bread was used as the standard, instead of glucose. After hundreds of food items were tested (generally in healthy volunteers), it was determined that refined grain products and potatoes have high GI values (causing high elevations in the blood sugar of these volunteers). Legumes and unprocessed grains have moderate GI values, and starchy fruits and vegetables have low values.

Since Dr. Jenkins and his group developed the GI in 1981, over 100 scientific studies have been conducted to examine the application of the GI to obesity, diabetes, and even cardio-vascular disease. Many popular nutrition books advocate diets based on items with a low GI. This advice is intuitively correct. If one eats food that causes the least elevations in blood-sugar levels, one would have a lower carbohydrate load and one should be better able to control one's diabetes. This idea was later endorsed by the Food and Agriculture Organization of the United Nations. But as you probably guessed, the typical Western diet still contains high concentrations of carbohydrates because it is based on potatoes, breads, and low-fat cereals.

Even though the diet based on food items with low GI values makes sense, the concept is not as simple as it first appears, and not everyone agrees about its usefulness. First, the GI was de-termined for each carbohydrate-containing food item—for example, rice, potato, and spaghetti. Most of us, however, eat mixed meals—not just rice or just potato or just spaghetti. We eat chips and fish, meat and potatoes, peanut butter and jelly, pork and beans, and so forth. Most of our meals contain multiple food items. Just look at our soups and gumbos to see how many ingredients are in one plate! The GI of the mixed meal has never been determined.

The second problem with relying on the GI for dieting purposes is that 90% of GIs have been determined in experiments with a small number of healthy, young volunteers—people who may digest, absorb, and respond to food items differently from people of middle age who have certain health problems. In fact, many older individuals and patients with diabetes digest and absorb food much more slowly than do younger and healthier people. Remember that each of us has a unique way of handling food—you are not your brother Tommy!

Third, the GI of a food item is influenced profoundly by its type, by its processing, and by its preparation. For example, the GI values of different types of rice vary by almost 100%! Similar differences have been found for different types of pasta, apples, and many other foods. Methods of food processing, including grinding, pressing, and rolling, affect the GI dramatically. So does the application of heat and moisture, as well as cooling and time of processing. All these steps can damage the outer layers of grains and the chemical composition of starches, thereby affecting significantly the GI of these foods.

Finally, the way a food is cooked also modifies its GI. The amount of heat used, the amount of water or sauce, the cooking time—all are important factors in modifying the GI of food items. In general, the more we heat, moisturize, grind, or press a starch-containing item, the higher the GI of this item is. The reason is that warmer, moister, and more finely ground food items are more easily digested and rapidly absorbed.

Attempting to design a low-GI diet, one could easily drown in the long list of GIs published in the 2002 "International Table of Glycemic Indices" in the *American Journal of Clinical Nutrition.* The list contains nearly 1,300 data entries! A better, much more practical solution is to limit carbohydrates in your diet, as outlined in my recommendations. If you want to lose weight, don't complicate your life by trying to identify low-GI food items. Instead, eliminate from your diet the main of-fenders: potatoes, pasta, and all sweet and baked goods. Enjoy your carbohydrates in fruits and vegetables (but avoid bananas, grapes, and corn).

## Dietary Fat

We consume two types of fat: cholesterol and fatty acids. The same cholesterol and fatty acids are also produced naturally in the body, but consumption of increased amounts of fat can greatly influence the overall concentrations of fat in the blood and in the bodily stores.

Cholesterol is absorbed from the gastrointestinal tract with the help of bile, which simply functions as a detergent to dissolve cholesterol. After being absorbed, cholesterol moves quickly into the liver. A large proportion of it is then released back into the gastrointestinal tract. Because of this efficient recycling system, it is very difficult to increase the levels of cholesterol in the blood by eating additional cholesterol. As a rule, people who have elevated cholesterol levels have a naturally elevated production of cholesterol in their bodies that they inherited from their parents.

Other fats are broken down in the gut (intestines) into single fatty acids. Not all fatty acids are created equal. They actually come in three varieties: saturated, monounsaturated, and polyunsaturated. *Saturated* means that every bond of every carbon atom in the fatty acid is connected with a different chemical group. When a single carbon atom of the fatty acid contains an extra available bond, the fatty acid is said to be *unsaturated*. When more than one unsaturated carbon atom is present in the molecule, the fatty acid is *polyunsaturated*.

Saturated fatty acids appear to be associated with heart and blood vessel disease. Unsaturated fatty acids, especially monounsaturated ones, appear to be protective against cardiovascular disease. Saturated fatty acids (known as "the bad fat," even though it has never been established in human beings whether saturated fat is really "bad") are

*Saturated fatty acids appear to be associated with heart and blood vessel disease. Unsaturated fatty acids, especially monounsaturated ones, appear to be protective against cardiovascular disease.*

present in meat, eggs, palm oil, and coconut oil. Polyunsaturated fatty acids are found in cold-water fish, soybeans, nuts, and canola oil. Monounsaturated fatty acids are contained in olive oil, canola oil, avocados, and nuts. The so-called Mediterranean diet is famous for its beneficial effect on the heart and its high content of monounsaturated fatty acids. Practically speaking, to eat healthfully, you should eat more fish than red meat and more olives, avocados, and olive oil than butter and eggs. Do not use palm or coconut oil. Make sure proteins are included in every meal or snack. Remember, fat and proteins frequently come together, as in eggs, fish, and nuts.

## Alcohol

First off, what do we do with alcohol? To drink or not to drink? For many of us, alcoholic beverages have become a part of life; if not a daily routine, then a social one. To have a beer, a glass of wine, or a cocktail is an integral part of social interactions, whether with our friends, relatives, or colleagues or even alone. But if your commitment to losing weight is genuine and serious—if you really, truly want to shed pounds—do not consume alcohol. Each and every gram of alcohol contains seven calories that will add to your caloric intake. More important, most alcoholic beverages contain a lot of carbohydrates, especially beer, sweet wines, and wine coolers. Beer and wine coolers are deadly to your diet. Furthermore, alcoholic beverages increase your appetite. Within minutes after ingestion, alcohol reduces blood-sugar levels and triggers a hunger signal to your brain. With food in front of you, you will inevitably eat more after having a drink or two than you would have with just a glass of seltzer. In patients with diabetes, alcohol may actually raise blood-sugar levels, worsening their control of their diabetes. Because it is so vital to your success, I wish to repeat my advice. If you are serious about your commitment to weight reduction or to a weight-maintenance program, avoid alcoholic drinks, by all means.

Having said this, I realize that, on occasion, you may find yourself in a situation where you simply cannot refuse an invitation to imbibe. If you are in such a predicament and if you find it hard to refuse a drink, I can offer you two options. The first is simply to ask for one glass of dry, nonsweet wine (preferably a red one) and to drink no more. Dry table wines contain fewer calories and carbohydrates and less alcohol than do other drinks. Your second option is to ask for a drink that you truly dislike and just touch it with your lips once or twice during the evening. You will save face, and no one will refill your glass!

As always, with drinking, one should be cognizant of the amount of alcohol consumed. For example, 3 oz of dry table wine contain sixty-eight calories, whereas a 12-oz can of beer contains 151 calories. But if you drink 12 oz of dry table wine, you will consume 272 calories (68 calories × 4 = 272 calories). Similarly, 1.5 oz of hard liquor contains 107 calories. *Please* do not drink 10 oz of hard liquor! Aside from your having consumed 740 calories, your evening may not end well.

## Eating Out

When you dine out, follow Draznin rules eight and nine. The eighth Draznin Rule is as follows: If you are overweight and are trying to lose weight, never, ever go to a restaurant that serves Asian food. The food there might be excellent, but if you have a problem with your weight and/or have diabetes, stay away. Practically all the items on the menu in these restaurants contain sugar, and a lot of it! Not good for a weight-reduction diet! The ninth Draznin Rule is as follows:

*The eighth Draznin Rule is as follows: If you are overweight and are trying to lose weight, never, ever go to a restaurant that serves Asian food.*

While dining out, order only grilled or broiled meat or fish—and never order anything that is deep-fried, pan-fried, or covered with sauces. If you are serious about losing weight, never order pasta, potatoes, or rice but only green and red vegetables. If your entrée comes with either potato or rice, eat as little as you possibly can and never more than *half* of your serving. Whenever possible, order an appetizer or a salad and split an entrée with your companion. When it comes to dessert, fresh fruit is your best option. However, if you have not eaten any carbohydrate at all, choose the least caloric dessert and split it with your dining partner.

*The ninth Draznin Rule is as follows: While dining out, order only grilled or broiled meat or fish—and never order anything that is deep-fried, pan-fried, or covered with sauces.*

In the restaurant, please talk to your waiter. Ask how large the portion is and whether you can share your entrée if it is too big. Find out how the food is prepared—broiled, fried, steamed, or sautéed. Can sauce or dressing be served on the side? Will the chef substitute side dishes? Don't be shy—some waiters love these questions. In their minds, the longer the preorder discussion, the greater the tip at the end of the meal. For you, the answers can be critical. For example, let us say tonight you fancy clams. Two ounces of steamed clams contain sixty calories and less than a gram of fat. In contrast, the same 2 oz of clams breaded and deep-fried contain 250 calories and 13 g of fat. Which one should you order? While reading the menu, go straight to fish dishes. If there is nothing there that you fancy, jump to poultry dishes as an option B. Finally, always ask your waiter not to bring complimentary bread. You waited four or five hours for your dinner, you can wait twenty more minutes without bread until your appetizer shows up.

Now, what do you do if you are invited to someone's house for dinner? If it is a good friend, call the person and share your dietary philosophy. Tell your friends that you can only eat grilled food and that you are trying to limit both fat and carbohydrate intake. Explain carefully what you mean and what food you will eat with pleasure and without restrictions. Most people will be very supportive.

If, on the other hand, you do not feel as though you can call and discuss your situation with your host, have a snack at home, about an hour before dinner, so you will not be hungry at the table. When you are not hungry, you are better able to control both your appetite and your choice of foods.

## Vitamins and Supplements

Vitamins are absolutely essential for many biochemical reactions within various cells. They help numerous enzymes carry out their appropriate functions. Deficiencies in vitamins readily impair these important functions, resulting in malfunctioning of different bodily systems. In extreme cases, vitamin deficiency can cause severe and even fatal disease. In a similar manner, frequently certain biochemical reactions in various cells require the presence of very specific minerals, such as magnesium, chromium, calcium, and others. Mineral deficiency can also cause significant impairment in bodily functions.

We obtain most vitamins and minerals from the foods we eat. Generally speaking, a normal diet of 2,000 calories or more, which includes meat, dairy products, fruits, and vegetables, contains sufficient vitamins and minerals and rarely, if ever, requires supplementation. In contrast, however, diets containing 1,200 calories or less do not supply adequate amounts of vitamins and minerals, and these should definitely be supplemented. Similarly, diets that selectively exclude certain food items, such as vegetarian diets or diets without fruits or vegetables, must be supplemented with vitamins and minerals.

Make sure you discuss your needs for vitamins and minerals with your doctor. My practical advice is that you take vitamin and mineral supplements, particularly iron and folate, if your diet contains fewer than 1,500 calories. If you are a vegetarian, you definitely need vitamins $B_2$ and $B_{12}$ as well as calcium, iron, and zinc. If you are over sixty-five, you may need calcium, selenium, and folate. In any event, you must have an informative conversation with your physician about vitamin and mineral supplements.

*Make sure you discuss your needs for vitamins and minerals with your doctor.*

Choose a multivitamin preparation that provides no more than 100% of the daily value ("% DV" is what is shown on the label) for all the vitamins and minerals included. You certainly do not want any of the side effects of excessive intake of some of these compounds. Only buy supplements that have the U.S.

Pharmacopeia (USP) symbol of quality on their label. Remember that most vitamins are better absorbed with food. However, calcium and iron may decrease the absorption both of each other and of other nutrients. They should be taken separately.

Finally, do not forget antioxidants. Most natural antioxidants are present in dark green and dark orange/red fruits and vegetables. The medicinal value of antioxidant vitamins, such as beta-carotene and vitamins C and E, has not been scientifically confirmed.

## Prescription and Over-the-Counter Medications

Diets themselves, particularly successful ones on which the dieter is losing weight, may have an impact on the effectiveness of some medications, and so may certain vitamins and minerals. Also, medications can alter the absorption and function of particular vitamins and minerals. Interactions can go either way, and your medications may suddenly become either more effective or less effective. In both cases, adjustments have to be made. That is why you must discuss this issue with your doctor as soon as you begin your dietary efforts.

## Cooking and Eating at Home

You can substantially reduce the number of calories you consume by changing your cooking habits, and without sacrificing the taste of your favorite dishes (or at least sacrificing very little!). The number-one rule is to buy proper ingredients, as described here. To begin with, the lower the caloric density of the items you buy, the fewer calories will end up on your plate and, eventually, in your stomach. The second rule is to always grill, broil, steam, or poach your food—never fry it. Here are a few other tips that should help you change the way you cook:

- Always trim all the fat from meat and remove the skin from poultry.
- Always substitute low-fat or nonfat versions of the items in the cooking recipes.
- Serve food from the kitchen, and never bring serving plates to the table. Going for seconds should not be made easy.
- Do not ever watch TV or read while eating. Focus your full attention on the amount of food you are consuming.
- Eat slowly. In fact, eat as slowly as you can. Do not take anything into your mouth until the previous mouthful of food is completely chewed and swallowed.
- Store food out of sight.
- Set aside time to prepare fresh vegetables in bulk, and store them until you use them.
- Do not skip a meal, particularly on a day when you are going to a social function. If you are hungry, you will most definitely overeat.
- Brush your teeth after each meal. The taste of the toothpaste should replace the taste of food.
- Finish your last meal of the day at least three hours before you go to bed.

## Grocery Shopping

Here is another critical element of my practical advice: Learn how to select your food in the grocery store. The tenth Draznin Rule is as follows: Never, ever buy any food item that contains more than 6 g of sugar per serving.

*The tenth Draznin Rule is as follows: Never, ever buy any food item that contains more than 6 g of sugar per serving.*

There is only one exception to this rule, and it is milk. Milk is the only allowable fluid that has calories and the only allowable product that contains more than 10 g of sugar (actually, 11 g per serving in fat-free milk). The most appropriate food choices should contain no more than 6 g of sugar, and the best choices should have fewer than 3 g of sugar.

Items with lower sugar content are there on the shelves; you just have to look for them. You must become a "smart shopper," committed to the Draznin Plan. Let us examine, for example, four Hormel ready-to-eat dinners: Meat Loaf with Tomato Sauce (6 g of saturated fat and 7 g of sugar), Grilled Chicken Breast with Teriyaki Sauce (1 g of saturated fat and 30 g of sugar), Beef Tips with Gravy (2.5 g of saturated fat and 3 g of sugar), and Turkey Breast with Gravy (1 g of saturated fat and 2 g of sugar). It is not too difficult to see which one should be included in the Draznin Plan. The turkey breast is the number-one choice, with beef tips earning second place.

What else is on your shopping list? If you like yogurt, you should know that Dannon 99% Fat Free yogurt contains 36 g of sugar. A fat-free yogurt has 17 g of sugar, and the Light'n Fit creamy yogurt contains only 10 g of sugar. When you come to the aisle where you find the English muffins, you will see some with 2 g of sugar (sourdough), 7 g of sugar (twelve-grain), and 11 g of sugar (cinnamon and raisin). My choice is clear (the sourdough), and so should yours be.

High sugar content is as bad as a high content of saturated fat. *Always read food labels, and never go shopping hungry.* We all know from our very own experience that when we are hungry, we buy food items that we will later regret. Always go to the market with a shopping list you have prepared at home. If you are driving to the store and discover that you don't have a shopping list, return home and prepare one. With a list, you

**Table 11.1 Nutrient Claims and Their Meanings**

| Term | Meaning |
| --- | --- |
| Calorie-free | Fewer than 5 calories per serving |
| Cholesterol-free | Fewer than 2 mg of cholesterol per serving and no more than 2 g of saturated fat per serving |
| Fat-free | Fewer than 0.5 g of fat per serving |
| Sugar-free | Fewer than 0.5 g of sugar per serving |
| Low-calorie | No more than 40 calories per serving |
| Low-cholesterol | No more than 20 mg of cholesterol and no more than 2 g of saturated fat per serving |
| Low-fat | No more than 3 g of fat per serving |
| Extra lean | No more than 5 g of fat, 2 g of saturated fat, and 95 mg of cholesterol per serving |
| Lean | Fewer than 10 g of fat, 4.5 g of saturated fat, and 95 mg of cholesterol per serving |
| Light or lite | One-third fewer calories or 50% less fat per serving than regular food |
| Reduced | 25% less fat per serving than regular food |

will buy only what you have preselected—only what you need. Without a list, you will buy on the spur of the moment, usually high-fat, high-carbohydrate items.

As you wander down the aisles examining the shelves, you must understand what the nutrient claims provided by the manufacturers really mean. Table 11.1 offers a partial list for your edification. As you can see, one must check labels carefully and understand "manufacturer jargon." Many items contain more calories, fat, and sugar than may appear to be the case from reading the label.

## Dairy Products

When you shop for dairy foods, remember that they are excellent sources of calcium, vitamin D, and protein. A cup of skim milk, for example, contains 8 g of protein. At the same time, there are today many "reduced-fat" dairy products on the market. As a rule, nonfat items have little taste, and many are outright unpleasant. In contrast, low-fat products taste almost as good as do our favorite nonreduced items. Unless you are on a very strict low-fat diet, you should still enjoy low-fat dairy products and not challenge your palate with tasteless nonfat substitutes.

Conversely, if you mix dairy products into recipes (for example, sour cream for salad dressing), the nonfat kinds will do just fine. By the way, instead of buying flavored yogurt, you might try mixing fresh fruit into plain yogurt—do your own flavoring, so to speak.

Finally, as an alternative to ice cream, fruit-containing sorbets are delicious, and they contain almost no fat and no added sugar.

## Meat

When shopping for meat, look for the leanest cuts: loin, leg, or round. If you are buying beef, choose the "select" grade over the "choice" grade as the former is the leaner. Overall, the leanest cuts of beef (when trimmed of fat before cooking) are eye-round, top-round, and sirloin steak. These cuts contain fewer than 7 g of fat. The leanest pork cut, with only 4 g of fat, is pork tenderloin. Trimmed boneless loin roast, boneless sirloin chop, and boneless loin chops contain fewer than 7 g of fat. In poultry, skinless chicken and turkey are low in fat, with white meat being leaner than dark meat. Always remember that "ground turkey" contains more fat than "ground turkey breast." Duck and goose are much higher in fat than are chicken and turkey.

## Soy

Soy, an excellent alternative source of protein, is becoming a mainstream product for many dieters. Soy products like tofu and tempeh take on the flavor of whatever sauce, marinade, or seasoning you decide to use with them. There are literally hundreds of delicious and varied recipes for the preparation of soy products. The main advantage of soy products for a weight-conscious consumer is their low content of both fat and carbohydrates. For example, Mori-Nu tofu (one of the best-tasting tofus, in my opinion) contains no fat and only a single gram of carbohydrate per 3-oz serving.

## Snacks

Unless you are slim and regularly exercise, avoid all snacks and candy bars. Most commercially available snacks are not just high in fat or high in carbohydrates—instead, they represent a mixture of both! Most snacks are low in proteins and low in moisture. They are basically designed *Avoid all snacks* for those who need an extra load of carbohydrates *and candy bars.* between bouts of moderate to strenuous exercise. If your goal is to lose weight, the best you can do is to lose any interest in snack bars.

Some people prefer nuts for snacks. Most nuts contain between 8% and 18% protein and 70%–90% unsaturated fat. They are usually free of cholesterol. Almonds are rich in calcium and fiber. Chestnuts are unique because they contain mainly carbohydrate and are low in fat. Pecans are among the highest in fat and lowest in protein. Macadamia nuts are sweet and creamy, and they have more fat and calories than do any other nuts. As a rule, an ounce of nuts contains 160–200 calories.

Fruit is another popular midmorning and midafternoon snack. Fruit can be fine if it is not overly sweet. Sweet fruits that contain large amounts of sugar can cause excessive release of insulin that will, in turn, precipitate the feeling of hunger thirty to sixty minutes after the snack. Almond or cashew butter, nonfat string cheese, tuna salad, chicken or turkey breast, avocado, or a few raw nuts are examples of better snacks than fruit.

Here is a list of food items you should not eat or drink if you are serious about losing weight:

- Asian food (unless homemade, without added sugar)
- Bananas (extremely high carbohydrate content)
- Beer
- Breaded meat or fish
- Candy
- Deep-fried food
- Dry fruit (very high sugar content)
- Grapes (almost pure sugar—glucose)
- Hamburger or hot-dog buns
- Mixed drinks
- Pasta
- Pizza
- Regular soda (a major culprit—high sugar content)
- Regular bread, rolls, bagels, and pastries
- Sauces (most contain sugar and high amounts of sodium)
- Sugar-coated baked food
- Sweet wine
- Watermelon (oh, how sweet it can be!)
- Anything that contains more than 3 g of saturated fat per serving

- Anything that contains more than 6 g of sugar per serving (except milk)

Here is a list of food items you should minimize in your diet if you are serious about losing weight:

- Cereals
- Dry table wine
- Low-calorie breads
- Potatoes
- Red meat
- Rice

Here are some basic rules for how to maintain your diet while eating out in a restaurant:

- No alcohol
- Meat or fish grilled or broiled only
- Meat portion no larger than the size of your palm
- Never anything fried, deep-fried, or breaded
- Low-calorie sauces and dressing only and served on the side
- No more than half a portion of the carbohydrate-containing sides, such as potatoes or rice
- For dessert (the best choice is to skip it, but you can order it if no carbohydrate-containing vegetables were consumed with your entrée), order frozen yogurt, light fruit pie, or fresh fruit
- Try to have an appetizer and split the entrée

As I stated in my introductory letter at the start of this book, to maintain a diet is not an easy task. In addition to your commitment, the diet must be comprised of items you like to eat and must not be too complicated. Finally, without increasing your energy expenditure, you still may fail to lose or maintain your reduced weight. It is the entire package, the Draznin Plan, that you should have in mind when you embark on a journey to change your lifestyle. The rules of appropriate hypocaloric dieting can be further summarized as follows:

1. Never eat, buy, or bring home anything that contains more than 6 g of sugar per serving (milk is the only exception).
2. Never eat, buy, or bring home anything that contains more than 2 g of saturated fat per serving.
3. Eat no more than six Draznin Calories per meal and no more than eighteen Draznin Calories per day.
4. Do three Draznin Miles a day.

*Chapter Twelve*

# My Own Personal Struggle to Prevent Diabetes

---

I am an average man—of an average size, that is. I am five feet nine inches tall and weigh 176 lb, which sets my body mass index (BMI) at 26. In order to get my BMI under the healthy ceiling of 25, I have to either drop my weight below 169 lb or grow an inch taller. Unfortunately, the latter is no longer an option and the former is very, very difficult to do. Realistically, my goal is to keep my BMI where it is now, at 26. At times, it was a bit greater; I once tipped the scale at 185 lb, the most I ever weighed. Most of the time, however, I've been reasonably successful in keeping my weight at around 174–176 lb.

I am not certain whether I inherited strong longevity genes from my parents. I hope I did. We will have to live and see. If I do have longevity genes, I hope to pass them on to my offspring. What I am certain about is that I have a strong family history of diabetes. Growing up, I was totally unaware of the medical history of my family. *I have a strong family history of diabetes.* Alongside a handful of pleasant memories that I retain from my childhood and adolescence is the recollection that I was always hungry ("A growing boy," my mother used to say) and always physically active, maybe even hyperactive ("This kid is a fountain of energy," my father used to add).

## A Growing Boy

Unencumbered by knowledge of nutrition and the dietary composition of food, I ate whatever I liked. Since my favorite dish was pasta, I ate a large plate of pasta every day. My mother used to prepare it for me as an after-school snack. Mainly, it was a plate of penne pasta, but it could be elbow, bow tie, egg-noodle, macaroni, or simple vermicelli. Pasta was my staple food—I could eat it several times a day, if it were available. In contrast, I never liked vegetables. I do not believe I ate a veg-etable until I turned 20 years old! By the same token, I loved ice cream. Chocolate ice cream was the best! Cold and creamy with fat and sugar added, it tasted delicious! I do not remember ever having enough of it. No matter how much ice cream I ate, I always wanted more.

No wonder I was on the chubby side of the growth curve on my pediatrician's chart. What saved me from becoming a real blob child was my love for athletic games: soccer, ice hockey, volleyball, team handball, short- and middle-distance running, long and high jump. I really loved it all. I was never among the best athletes but frequently made it to the second-tier teams and occasionally to the varsity level. Most importantly, I loved the game itself much more than the outcome of a given match or meet. Once I played goalie on a soccer team, and we lost 5 to 1 to another team. My teammates were crushed, but I was very happy with my performance. "If it were not for my outstanding play," I told them after the game, "the score would have been 10 to 1." I made quite a few great saves, I thought.

It was only in medical school that I learned the medical history of my family, finding out that my maternal grandfather died from complications of diabetes. He had gangrene of his left foot, refused amputation, and succumbed to sepsis (overwhelming blood infection) within a few weeks. Several years later, when my mother and her younger brother were diagnosed with type 2 diabetes, I realized that this disease is within striking distance of me as well.

As we have discussed on numerous occasions elsewhere in this book, realization alone does not guarantee, and does not even suggest that one will attempt or contemplate attempting, making a change. The truth be known—I did very little initially. The realization had to sink in. I don't know how long it took in terms of time, but I remember growing two full sizes of clothing before I made my first change.

## Initiating Dietary Change

This change was to give up desserts. Not easy but not too difficult either. The second step was to take up jogging on a more regular basis. I began with about twenty minutes a day, building it up to thirty minutes, trying to do it at least five days a week. I jogged at the nearby high school track—four laps equal one mile. I tried to squeeze in between eight and twelve laps. Within four months I lost one clothing size and felt very encouraged.

But the second size did not want to leave me. It was nagging and teasing me for almost two years, until I made another step—practically eliminating my favorite pasta from my diet and reducing the amounts of carbohydrates I ate. This is when I added vegetables (salads) to my diet. Amazingly, I found them just fine—very tasty, that is. I realized I loved spinach salad, Greek salad, Caesar salad, and fancy salads with fruit and nuts. I guess I did not know what I was missing!

But salads aside, omitting pasta and reducing breads was probably the most important step at that point. My weight was coming down again. Slowly but surely. Somewhere around the same time, everyone in my family began avoiding high-fat items, switching to either reduced-fat or no-fat food items. We began buying nonfat milk, low-fat cream cheese, low-fat yogurts, low-fat meat. Our eating habits began to change. I must tell you, after you remove fatty products from your diet for a year or so, they no longer taste good and, in fact, grease becomes repulsive. New habits not only settle in, but they also protect you from your previous habits. A new lifestyle is now dominant.

It is harder to get away from smaller things—a candy, a cookie, a piece of chocolate, a scoop of ice cream—particularly when they are in your cupboard and your freezer. You open the door and they smile at you—take me, take me, I am right here! But one must learn to deal with them as well. The most important rule is to not buy them and never to bring them home. When you open your refrigerator and the only thing that looks back out at you is an English cucumber, you will not gain weight. At work, you might ask your coworkers not to bring sweets to the office. Most would agree.

*When you open your refrigerator and the only thing that looks back out at you is an English cucumber, you will not gain weight.*

## Finding the Right Exercise Program

Selecting an exercise program was not as easy as I thought. Initially, probably being enamored with the European and South American soccer stars and remembering fondly my childhood experience, I decided to try "my foot" at this game. I envisioned playing games on the lush carpet of local parks on cool mornings or late afternoons. The feel of being a part of a team was also appealing. Finally, I was under the impression that the players run (when the ball is next to you) and rest (when the ball is on the opposite side of the field) intermittently. I found an adult co-ed league and signed up without hesitation. I was forty-five years old, probably the oldest member of the team. I was proud of having been as active and as vigorous as any other member of the squad. At practices we ran, kicked the ball, headed it hard, and navigated around red cones.

The team, however, did not have a bona fide goalie. A few people tried but either didn't like it or did not have the quick reaction speed necessary to play this position. The coach seemed to be convinced I was the best candidate for the job. I didn't mind. I'd played this position before. To me, the competition between the goalie and the striker shooting at the goal looked like a duel, a "cat and mouse" play. The striker seemed to have an advantage—the goal is wide and difficult to defend. The key for the goalie, as I quickly found out, was to assume the correct position, to always be in the way of the ball, to make the shooting angle for the striker as difficult as possible. I liked my new position and was ready to play. The league's games started in two weeks. There was one thing, however, that I did not realize.

During one of the games, a long ball was kicked toward my goal. A striker from the opposite team, a young man about half my age and of about my body size, ran to the ball and jumped high in the air, trying to head it to the goal. I ran from the opposite direction and jumped high, trying to intercept the ball or at least to deflect it. We collided in the air. Two bodies bumped one another and fell on the ground. I guess I touched the ball with my stretched arm and it sailed out of bounds. Let me tell you, when the bones of a forty-five-year-old man collide with the bones of a twenty-five-year-old, the impact is not equal. The young striker got off the ground as if he had bounced off a soft mattress. I couldn't move for quite a while. The pain in my neck, shoulders, and low back was excruciating. The coach and other players carried me off the field and placed me under a tree, still stiff as a board. Another fifteen minutes passed before I was able to stand up. My soccer career ended with a great save and a bruised body that recovered only after three or four weeks. Luckily, I didn't break anything, and wisely I moved to another form of exercise.

Taking up tennis was my next attempt in developing habitual exercise. What a great game! It looks much easier than it really is. The learning curve in one's late forties and early fifties is steeper than I imagined. I felt as though I was spending much more time running to pick up balls than playing. Finding a suitable partner was also a problem. Most people played better than I and avoided my invitations. With others, I constantly had a hard time scheduling a match. The times convenient to them were frequently inconvenient to me and vice versa. So the idea of tennis had to be replaced with another.

At some point I signed up with a local hiking club, a wonderful group of the most cheerful people I had met in years. The club had a schedule of weekly hikes broken down by degree of difficulty, and members would select from the list. I learned fairly quickly that what they call a "moderate" hike represents a difficult hike for me. Instructors tended to underestimate the degree of difficulty and overestimate our ability. The most significant problem, however, was having to commit to weekly hikes on the weekends. This meant having to put family and frequently work obligations on the back burner. As a result, even though I loved to hike, the club proved to be an impractical solution.

I went back to individual walking and jogging. I did not need any partners and did not need to adjust my time to fit someone else's schedule. I could do it piecemeal—a short jog in the morning and a longer walk in the afternoon. I could do it any time and place. Jogging and walking became the exercise of choice.

*Jogging and walking became the exercise of choice.*

As I was getting older, it became more and more difficult to squeeze two or three miles into my daily twenty- or thirty-minute jog. I began pondering what is more important—to finish three miles or to be in motion for thirty minutes. Fortunately, the natural course of events had dictated the proper answer. With time, going by distance and finishing three miles required more time than the allotted thirty minutes. In addition, it made me much more tired not only during and immediately after the run but also on the next day. The effect on my weight and on my vigor remains very strong if I exercise by time regardless of distance. The concept of the Draznin Mile was born, that ten-minute jog or twenty-minute walk that is equal to one Draznin Mile—simple and powerfully effective. I can say this with certainty because, as you have learned from this chapter, the Draznin Plan works even for its inventor!

## Chapter Thirteen

# Case Studies and a Treatment Plan for Mr. K.

---

## Ms. Elizabeth E.

Ms. Elizabeth E., a forty-eight-year-old self-employed writer, was the mother of two children and had no health problems, except for being overweight and having type 2 diabetes. Ms. E. was five feet five inches tall and weighed 174 lb. Her body mass index (BMI) was 29. Ms. E. worked from home, and she was extremely disciplined about her writing and editing assignments. She allocated three hours in the morning and three hours in the afternoon to be at her desk. She also spent two hours a day reading. Aside from her usual household chores, she was not involved in any "extracurricular" physical activity.

During her second pregnancy, Ms. E.'s physician detected elevated blood-sugar levels. That was sixteen years before she came to see me. At that time, she was treated with three premeal injections of insulin per day. After delivery, her blood-sugar levels normalized and insulin was discontinued. She did not lose much weight after her pregnancy and, in fact, continued to gain weight over the next five to six years.

Eight years later, at the age of forty, she was diagnosed with overt diabetes, type 2. She was started on oral antidiabetic medications and advised to follow a low-fat diet, with 55%–60% carbohydrates derived mainly from complex carbohydrates and fiber. At the time, Ms. E. believed it would be easy to adhere to these new dietary recommendations, particularly in light of the fact that she had always turned to pasta as a source of healthy carbohydrates and her entire household loved pasta dishes. Pasta is easy to cook and, with various sauces, provides great variety in taste. But her diabetes remained poorly controlled.

Because Ms. E.'s blood sugar was continuously above 200 mg/dl and her glycosylated hemoglobin ($HbA_{1C}$) hovered around 9%, her doctor placed her on two injections of insulin a day. Over the next couple of months, her doctor increased the dose of insulin; and when Ms. E. came to see me, she was taking forty-eight units of insulin in the morning and thirty-six units before dinner. Her diabetes improved somewhat, with blood sugar declining to 150 mg/dl and $HbA_{1C}$ to 8%. However, after that, she gained almost eighteen pounds, and that generated in her a lot of anxiety, frustration, and unhappiness.

Ms. E. realized that, after her insulin injections, she had to eat in order to prevent low blood sugar—the so-called insulin reaction. To deal with weight gain, Ms. E. began skipping insulin injections, first occasionally and then on a regular basis. When she came to see me, she was not taking her insulin on Tuesdays and Thursdays, in an attempt to eat less on those days. She had not disclosed this to her previous physician, and when I examined her, her $HbA_{1C}$ was 9.4%, reflecting almost constantly elevated blood-sugar levels. Instead of exercising,

*To deal with weight gain, Ms. E. began skipping insulin injections, first occasionally and then on a regular basis.*

Ms. E. decided to increase her physical activity by spending about two hours a day taking care of her beautiful garden.

### Discussion

Ms. E. was an intelligent woman who had been truly and conscientiously trying to follow the recommendations she had received from her doctor. She wanted to know more about her condition, and for a long time she adhered faithfully to the prescribed regimen. It was a failure of the therapeutic program that resulted in her frustration and poor compliance in taking her insulin. Eventually, her fear of gaining weight prevailed over the necessity of controlling her diabetes. Unfortunately, in this regard, Ms. E. is not alone. Several major studies have clearly documented significant weight gain in patients receiving insulin to control their diabetes. Certainly, taking increasing doses of insulin will eventually keep blood-glucose levels in check, but there is a price to pay. And patients pay this price with pounds of gained weight.

I asked Ms. E. to write down, honestly and meticulously, everything she ate during the next three days. She did, and we reviewed the list of food items that made their way into her diet. Her dietary recall revealed that she was consuming an average of 3,100 calories per day. That was clearly too much. To lose weight, she would have to consume about one-half this amount daily.

We designed a low-carbohydrate diet, with a minimal amount of saturated fat and reduced cholesterol. She began a hypocaloric diet of 1,600 calories per day. We also reduced her insulin dose by half, and she started a walking program, beginning at twenty minutes twice a day.

The results were very impressive. Ms. E. lost eight pounds in two weeks, her blood-sugar levels decreased to 120 mg/dl, and we further reduced her insulin dose. The plan is for her to stay on her 1,600-calorie diet, build up her exercise tolerance to three Draznin Miles a day, and discontinue insulin. At that time, she may or may not require other antidiabetic medications.

## Mr. Frederick D.

Mr. Frederick D. had a very different problem. He was a forty-two-year-old loan officer with a local bank and had type 1 diabetes. He was diagnosed at fifteen years old. Ever since, he had been treated with insulin injections as insulin is the only therapy for patients with type 1 diabetes. At the time he came to see me, he was administering three insulin injections to himself each day.

Mr. D. had never been advised to keep to a particular diet. Instead, he had been taught to count carbohydrates in his diet and to adjust his insulin dose accordingly in order to cover his carbohydrate load. He had followed this advice for twenty-seven years. He did it very efficiently, having reached a certain degree of perfection in carbohydrate counting. He could look at his meals and assess the number of carbohydrates almost instantaneously. Then, he would give himself a single unit of insulin for every 12 g of carbohydrates in his meal. Two years before, he had undergone laser therapy on both eyes, for retinal problems. A year later, he had an elevated blood pressure of 150/105 mm Hg and was placed on antihypertensive medication.

A month before he came to see me, laboratory evaluation revealed that his kidney function was significantly impaired.

He was told that within the next three to five years he would probably require either dialysis or kidney transplantation.

### Discussion

Twenty-seven years of diabetes had finally damaged Mr. D.'s eyes and kidneys. Though laser therapy for eye problems has saved the sight of millions of patients with diabetes, kidney disease remains a grave complication of the illness. Approximately 40% of patients with type 1 diabetes end up developing kidney failure. Many require dialysis, and many undergo kidney transplantation. Recent advances in the treatment of elevated blood pressure have reduced the rate of kidney failure in patients with diabetes, but it remains a colossal problem for these people and for the health-care system in general.

*Approximately 40% of patients with type 1 diabetes end up developing kidney failure.*

Major clinical studies have shown indisputably that better and tighter control of diabetes delays and prevents the development of these complications. Unfortunately, some patients, even those with excellent control of their diabetes, can still develop complications. We do not know why this is, but conceivably a certain genetic makeup may predispose these individuals to develop complications.

On a side note, I strongly disagree with the philosophy of ignoring diet and allowing a youngster to eat anything and everything and simply take more insulin to cover extra carbohydrates and extra calories. A number of diabetologists, dietitians, and psychologists believe that children and adolescents with diabetes should not be placed on dietary restrictions as these restrictions may have an adverse psychological effect. On the contrary, young patients with type 1 diabetes show tremendous and early psychological maturity. This is true not only for patients with diabetes but also for young patients with other serious or chronic illnesses. With appropriate support, it is my opinion that these children and young adults would gladly embrace the best approach to their conditions. And my approach to all patients with diabetes is to instill a firm commitment to diet therapy.

Back to Mr. D. Another point of vital importance was his elevated blood pressure (hypertension). Maintaining normal blood pressure is probably the single most important element in the treatment of diabetic patients with even mild hypertension. We now recognize that aggressive treatment of high blood pressure in patients with diabetes prolongs their lives, delays eye and kidney complications, and prevents heart attacks and stroke. A patient with diabetes should never have a blood pressure level greater than 130/85 mm Hg. Preferably, it should be less than 125/80 mm Hg. It was imperative for both Mr. D. and his physician to do everything and anything possible to reduce Mr. D.'s blood pressure to desirable levels.

I recommended that Mr. D. eliminate sugar, sweets, and baked goods from his diet immediately. I also designed a diet with low protein because his kidneys could no longer handle a significant protein load. The diet was also low in cholesterol and saturated fat. I would adjust his insulin intake weekly so as to find the optimal dose to control his diabetes. I began aggressive treatment of his hypertension, with both medications and meditation therapy. Finally, I checked his blood-lipid levels and recommended a lipid-lowering medication as well. Our hope was to delay the progression of his kidney disease, which was still very much an attainable goal, even in the presence of his already impaired kidney function.

And what about exercise? What about the three Draznin Miles for Mr. D.? At that time, he had to be extremely cautious with his exercise program. Strenuous exercise could further damage his kidney function. I preferred to stabilize his diabetes, to control his blood pressure, and then to perform a stress test. That would give us a reasonable assessment of the ability of his heart to handle an exercise load. Only at that point would I feel comfortable designing an exercise program for Mr. D.

Now, after we have discussed in detail the role of diet and exercise in weight reduction and weight maintenance, we should be able to give very specific recommendations to many other individuals with obesity and diabetes. I wish to present to you several case studies, examples from my clinical practice, and ask you, the reader, to participate with me in the decision-making process. I want to ensure not only that you read my book for its general educational value but also that you derive from it specific information that will be important in helping you address your own concerns with a clearer understanding of them.

*I want to ensure not only that you read my book for its general educational value but also that you derive from it specific information that will be important in helping you address your own concerns with a clearer understanding of them.*

The examples I offer to your attention should mirror some of the problems you might have, and they should help you solidify the knowledge you have gained from this book. I hope these case studies will also reinforce the notion that every person is different and that advice should be individualized, as much as possible. At the end of this exercise, we will design a very specific program for Mr. Jeffrey K., who is still sitting in my office awaiting answers.

## Case Study 1

Jason P., age twelve, came to see me because of a recent weight gain of approximately eighteen pounds. Even though Jason had grown about four inches over the previous summer and fall, an eighteen-pound weight gain rightly alarmed his parents, who brought Jason to my office. Jason's father was an engineer with a cable company, and his mother worked as a billing clerk for a group of physicians. Jason had grown up normally, with minimal medical problems. Over the previous year, he had become very involved with his computer and now spent almost all his free time in front of his PC. Though his parents were very proud of his ability to write computer programs and design sophisticated Web pages, they were concerned with his recent weight gain.

For breakfast, Jason usually had a glass of orange juice and a blueberry muffin. He would have a bag of chips and a can of regular Coke at school, and he would eat about two servings of macaroni and cheese when he arrived home from school. He would then eat again, at 7:00 PM, this time dinner with his family. The meal usually consisted of things like chicken with mashed potatoes or pizza. Jason would drink another can of regular Coke at the dinner table. A large-sized bag of corn chips and a Coke were always present at his computer desk, and he wouldn't even notice how many chips he ate at his computer.

**Question**. What should Jason do to prevent further weight gain and possibly lose excess weight in the near future?

**Answer**. Clearly, the computer had consumed Jason to the point that he had neither the time nor the desire to be involved in any physical activity. At the same time, his diet was extremely rich in carbohydrates. On this diet and without exercise, Jason was about to join the increasing ranks of obese children and young adults.

Before it was too late, his parents should convince Jason (or lead him, by example) to allocate some time in his daily routine for physical activities: walking, biking, playing basketball, swimming—anything but sitting in front of a PC monitor. Dietary habits would also have to be altered. Muffins, macaroni, pizza, and regular Coke—all must go. Vegetables, fruit, noncaloric drinks, and nonfat meat and poultry would have to be introduced into his diet. In order to place a twelve-year-old on a diet, all members of the household would have to change their dietary habits. It was absolutely mandatory for Jason to reverse his course toward obesity.

**Question.** For which one of the following four twelve-year-olds is a macaroni-and-cheese dinner *not* an appropriate choice?

a. A very active twelve-year-old boy who also plays soccer every day.
b. A normal-weight twelve-year-old boy who spends most of the day in front of his computer.
c. A normal-weight twelve-year-old girl who is a member of a competitive swim team.
d. A normal-weight twelve-year-old girl recovering from surgery for a broken leg.

The answer is b. All four children eat an unrestricted diet, making it very likely that the sedentary child who spends most of his day in front of a computer monitor consumes more than he spends. This sedentary youngster will quickly become overweight on a high-carbohydrate and high-fat diet. The girl recovering from surgery will have to adjust her diet when recovery is complete.

## Case Study 2

Ms. Marianne Z., a five-foot seven-inch woman weighing 185 lb, worked as a paralegal in a busy law office. She was thirty-five years old and had two children, ages five and seven. She had gained twenty pounds after the birth of her first child and over thirty pounds during and after her second pregnancy. Her thyroid-function tests were normal, and she did not have diabetes. Ms. Z. loved sweets and pastries, and she prepared a lot of sweet food items for her family. Pancakes with honey, cinnamon rolls, and Belgian waffles were her favorite breakfast foods. She had read that fatty food is bad, and she was trying conscientiously to buy low-fat items. She loved to bake and was proud of her culinary skills. She stayed busy at work and at home, but she was not involved in any structured exercise program.

**Question**.  What should Ms. Z. do to initiate weight loss?

**Answer**.  The very first thing Ms. Z. needed to do was to begin a hypocaloric diet. She had to eat less. She had to consume fewer calories than she expended. This was unquestionably the number-one rule for her success.

Ms. Z would have to change the nature of the food she ate, the way she cooked, and the food items she purchased. Many so-called low-fat foods contain excessive amounts of sugar and other carbohydrates that are not good for weight loss. Among her immediate steps, Ms. Z. had to switch herself and the entire

*Many so-called low-fat foods contain excessive amounts of sugar and other carbohydrates that are not good for weight loss.*

family to noncaloric beverages, change her breakfast routine, and eliminate 90% of her baking. Without these steps, she would never be successful in losing, or even maintaining, her weight. Subsequently, she would have to find time for three Draznin Miles a day.

**Question.** What is the most appropriate breakfast choice for a five-foot seven-inch woman weighing 185 lb?

a. One egg over easy, one slice of whole wheat toast, one unsweetened grapefruit.
b. One pancake with honey, a glass of orange juice.
c. One cinnamon roll with marmalade, coffee with skim milk.

The answer is a. This is the only choice that minimizes the intake of carbohydrates. Choices b and c would fit a high-carbohydrate diet and would be highly inappropriate for an obese woman.

## Case Study 3

Mr. Dwayne J. was a forty-two-year-old sales representative who was six feet tall and weighed 195 lb. He traveled extensively within the western United States, staying in hotels and eating out with his clients and colleagues. During the previous four years, he had gained twenty-five pounds. He had mild pain in his knees that limited his ability to walk, which he actually liked to do but for which he could find little time. Recently, his blood pressure had risen to 140/95 mm Hg.

He knew about some "minor" problem with his cholesterol, but he didn't remember what exactly it was. He was otherwise healthy. His father had died of a heart attack at the age of fifty-nine.

**Question**. What should Mr. J. do to lose weight?

**Answer**. At the age of forty-two, with elevated blood pressure, probably elevated cholesterol, and a family history of a heart attack, Mr. J. had first to undergo an exercise stress test and then we would reevaluate his lipid levels. Provided he was ready for it, Mr. J. ought immediately to start an exercise program, building up to three Draznin Miles a day. Considering his knee pain, stationary biking or swimming might be his best options. He should also start a hypocaloric diet, eliminating high-fat and high-carbohydrate items. His new diet should consist of grilled meat and fish, with vegetables. It goes without saying that he should stop drinking alcohol either before or with his meals.

**Question**. Which one of these four 195-lb individuals should not eat a 900-calorie shrimp-and-pasta dinner?

   a. A five-foot eleven-inch college student competing for a spot on a football team.
   b. A five-foot seven-inch thirty-five-year-old former high school and college wrestler who works out and jogs three miles daily.
   c. A five-foot nine-inch thirty-nine-year-old lawyer who is trying to lose weight.
   d. A six-foot two-inch, thirty-four-year-old auto mechanic who is on a low-fat diet.

The answer is c. A high-carbohydrate meal would not be beneficial to a sedentary person who is trying to lose weight. It might, however, be appropriate for an athletic person who is involved in a regular, more than moderate exercise program.

I hope you have answered all these questions correctly. Let us now return to Mr. Jeffrey K., our protagonist and my patient, waiting to hear my advice regarding his weight, diabetes, and high blood pressure. Without becoming engulfed in many small details, for the purpose of our discussion I submit to you that my advice will be concerned with four general areas: diet, exercise, lifestyle, and medications. Because the "medication" topic is too specific and highly professional, it is clearly beyond the scope of this book. Let us put it aside and discuss my recommendations for diet, exercise, and lifestyle in great detail.

First there is a sensible and realistic hope for Mr. K. Two large studies have confirmed what many of us already knew from our individual experiences: Appropriate diet and exercise prevented the development of diabetes in almost 60% of people participating in these studies. In a Finnish study, 172 middle-aged and overweight men and 350 women achieved, on average, a 4-kg (8.8-lb) weight loss in one year. They maintained a 3.5-kg (7.7-lb) weight loss during the second year of the study as well. At the end of the second year, the risk of these individuals' developing diabetes was reduced by 58%!

> *Two large studies have confirmed what many of us already knew from our individual experiences: Appropriate diet and exercise prevented the development of diabetes in almost 60% of people participating in these studies.*

A second study was conducted in the United States. A large clinical trial, called the Diabetes Prevention Program, enrolled 3,234 participants with impaired glucose tolerance, a condition that commonly leads to diabetes. On a low-fat diet and with exercise of 150 minutes each week, these individuals also reduced their risk of developing diabetes by 58%!

Splendid, wonderful, and encouraging news for Mr. K.! His chances of winning his battle with his early diabetes are greater than 50%!

## Diet

Mr. K. weighs 230 lb and is six feet tall. Because his ideal body weight is approximately 180 lb, he has a long way to go. If we establish a fifty-pound weight reduction as our initial goal, we will most likely fail. This goal is simply unrealistic at this point. We should be much more modest and set our goal at a twenty-pound weight loss within the first year, getting Mr. K. down to 210 lb. This will be a loss of approximately 8% of his starting weight. If he is successful in attaining this goal and maintaining his reduced weight, we might revise our goals and expectations; but for now, this 8% weight loss seems to be a realistic and achievable goal.

The very first thing I want Mr. K. to do is to keep a precise list of what he eats—a diary, or "dietary recall," as it is called. Whatever food item makes its way to Mr. K.'s mouth has to be recorded in his food diary. This is the only way to objectively monitor what he eats, to analyze his caloric intake, and to make appropriate adjustments. After a certain period of time under my guidance, he will learn to make these adjustments on his own. Some people object to keeping such a list, arguing that this exercise focuses them on their problems, instead of allowing them to live free of them. I believe that maintaining this list strengthens our commitment to weight-reduction goals. After all, we are on a lifelong mission to change the way we eat and the way we live.

I will also ask Mr. K. to eliminate from his home and from his diet margarine, candies, pastries, flour, sugar, cereals, sour cream, whipped cream, pasta, beer, and all other items that contain more than 6 g of sugar and/or 2 g of saturated fat per serving. I also want Mr. K. and his wife to spend an hour, twice a week, in their favorite grocery store, reading and comparing labels of various food items—those that they used to buy and those that they will be buying from now on. They must understand what they are purchasing.

I invited Ms. K. to accompany her husband to his next appointment with me. She is an integral member of our team, and her support, understanding, and cooperation are absolutely critical.

Table 13.1 is a sample menu that the three of us decided would be acceptable for Mr. K. A number of variations can be introduced to this basic menu, but the goal remains the same—to design a hypocaloric diet containing no more than eighteen Draznin Calories a day (between 1,500 and 1,800 calories) with moderate amounts of carbohydrates.

## Exercise

Jeffrey K. is a very sedentary man, but he does not have any other health problems aside from his recently diagnosed diabetes and mild hypertension. He is also over thirty-five years of age, and I would like to see a normal exercise stress test before recommending an exercise program to him, even one as simple as three Draznin Miles. Once the stress test clears him for an exercise program, he can easily start his way to the three Draznin Miles a day program. He can accomplish this by walking

**Table 13.1  Sample Menu for Mr. K**

**Breakfast**

One soft- or hard-boiled egg (can be pan-fried with a nonstick spray)
One slice of whole wheat bread or toast (preferably low-calorie bread)
½ cup of berries or 2 slices of melon
Water, tea, or coffee

**Midmorning Snack**

Cup of tea with 1 small apple, 5 almonds, or a slice of cheese

**Lunch**

Big bowl of salad, with low-fat dressing
Grilled chicken, turkey breast, or tuna
Water, tea, or diet soda

**Midafternoon Snack**

8–10 peeled small carrots
1 apple or pear
Water, diet soda, or tea

**Dinner**

Large salad with low-fat dressing
Grilled meat, poultry, or fish
Steamed or stir-fried vegetables
1 cup of berries or 2 slices of melon or watermelon
Sugarless fruit popsicle
Water, tea, or coffee

ten minutes away from his home and ten minutes back, twice a day. I want him to do this for three weeks and then increase his walking distance to fifteen minutes each way. This would translate into an hour a day of walking! This is a great goal for the next couple of months. The magic three Draznin Miles a day are within his reach.

Meanwhile, I want Mr. K. to buy a pair of new and comfortable walking shoes and a pedometer. Realizing that the goal is to take at least 10,000–11,000 steps daily, he should know where he stands right now and the progress he will be making on his way to the goal. I firmly believe that even a small investment will offer a huge boost to his motivation.

## Lifestyle

Changing his diet and embarking on a walking program are already great improvements in Mr. K.'s lifestyle. But we want more. Fortunately, he does not smoke, and he drinks only minimal amounts of wine. I do not believe it will be difficult for him to abstain from alcohol. I want Mr. and Ms. K. to find out what kinds of meditation and yoga classes are available in their community. I want them to visit some of these programs and speak to the instructors. We plan to discuss their findings about a month from now, when they are somewhat adjusted to their new diet and exercise routine.

We shake hands, and Mr. K. leaves my office. He will return in a week (after his exercise test) with Ms. K. and an initial report on his progress. He will certainly bring the list of food items he has eaten during the week. We will recheck his blood-sugar level and blood pressure and spend some time together. We will have taken the first two steps on his long road to success.

We come at last to conclusions, to the summary of my thoughts. You are now the master of the Draznin Plan. Remember the third leg of the Draznin Plan's foundation—the three-legged stool—your personal commitment. Now that you know everything else, your personal commitment has become a key to your success. Do not get discouraged by temporary setbacks. You are only human—you fall off the wagon, so get back in as soon as you can. Time flies fast as it is, you cannot afford to lose extra days and weeks. It is not that overwhelmingly difficult. After all, you have learned to brush your teeth, wash your hands as well as fruit and vegetables, greet your neighbors, and thank people who do something nice for you. I am absolutely convinced you can build another habit—to do three Draznin miles a day and avoid sweets and fats in your diet.

One of the greatest improvements in human health came with the realization that water must be boiled before use. This one simple (as we now know) step saved millions of lives. Unfortunately and sadly, there are still places in the world where this is not done. But we are beyond this. Our next major battle is self-indulgence—too much food, too little effort. I believe that once we understand this, we can deal with the problem. My plan does. With your commitment, you will be able to do it. Try it and write to me—Boris.Draznin@uchsc.edu. Good luck! It was a great pleasure writing my plan for you.

# Recommendations Based on Ten Draznin Rules of Life

*Science is the orderly arrangement of what, at the moment, seem
to be the facts.*

Anonymous

## Recommendation 1
Three Draznin Miles and fewer than eighteen Draznin Calories
a day are the keys to your successful fight with obesity and
diabetes.

## Recommendation 2
Select a knowledgeable doctor who has both the interest and
the time to discuss your lifestyle problems with you.

## Recommendation 3
Develop a set of reasonable goals, and tackle them one by one.

## Recommendation 4
Do not stay on a very low–calorie diet for more than ten days.
Rather, always be on a hypocaloric diet that has been devel-
oped to meet your goals.

## Recommendation 5

Always stay on a low-carbohydrate diet, unless your body mass index is under 25 and you do at least six Draznin Miles a day.

## Recommendation 6

Exclude saturated fat from your diet, but do not be afraid of mono- and polyunsaturated fats. Remember that a Mediterranean diet based on these fats is both healthy and tasty.

## Recommendation 7

Never eat or drink anything that contains more than 6 g of sugar per serving.

## Recommendation 8

Remember that, at every stage of your life, you are personally responsible for at least 90% of its quality.

## Recommendation 9

He who would eat the kernel must crack the nut. You must have a lifelong commitment to your lifestyle choices. It is never too late to start your commitment.

## Recommendation 10

Never forget Recommendation 1!

# Frequently Asked Questions

P eople in general, and my patients are not an exception, always have questions about their health. I do everything possible to encourage my patients not only to generate these questions but to bring them to my attention. Their questions reflect the individuality of their problems, and I hope my answers boost their confidence in, adherence to, and compliance with their treatment plans. What follow are typical questions my patients ask, followed by short answers that might be helpful to you. I will also tell you how to contact me and make use of other sources to help answer questions and concerns you have.

**Question 1**. I started on your program about three months ago, and I am still doing fairly well with the dietary part. However, it's the walking part that gives me trouble. I've built up my walking program to twenty minutes a day, and I just don't seem to have time either in the morning or in the evening to increase my exercise. I leave home early, return about 600,. we eat dinner at 6:30 or 7:00, and after dinner I am too tired to go out. I watch TV for about an hour and then read in bed for about twenty to thirty minutes. Do you have any suggestions as to how I can deal with my problem?

**Answer 1**. I understand that you have a long workday and find it difficult to squeeze in more exercise. We can deal with this in several ways. First, there is a wonderful program developed at the University of Colorado Health Science Center under the direction of Dr. James Hill. Participants are asked to wear a pedometer, a little gizmo that is worn on the belt and counts the number of steps one makes. After a week, a staff member calculates the average number of steps the participant did daily and asks him or her to add 2,000 steps every day. These 2,000 steps can be made at any time during the day. They can come from walking an extra flight of stairs, parking your car farther away in the parking lot and walking the extra distance, or making another circle around the park. The 2,000 steps represent about one mile, and adding them to your daily walking regimen can go a long way toward your three Draznin Miles a day.

The second way of finding time to exercise is to use the time you watch TV. This way is a bit more expensive. You should purchase a treadmill, place it in front of your TV, and use it while watching your favorite program. Personally, if I watch a sporting event, I do it only while walking on my treadmill.

**Question 2**. I have noticed that lately both my husband and I feel extremely anxious about several things in our lives. things like job security, pension funds, our teenage children, and our elderly parents. Every time I worry about one of these things, I feel hungry, I eat, and, not surprisingly, I gain weight. Is there a relationship between anxiety and weight gain?

**Answer 2**. Very much so, even though no one knows the exact nature of this relationship. Conceivably, chemical and/or hormonal imbalance in the brain can be the culprit. Brain cells misfire, disconnect, lose inhibitory control, and become incompetent in regulating the sense of satiety. At the same time, anxiety can be accompanied by increased output of adrenaline, which can change the levels of glucose in the blood and, consequently, the levels of insulin and the sensation of hunger.

Let me share with you a story about my patient Mr. Zi. Mr. Zi is a private investigator who also repossesses automobiles on behalf of lenders when people default on their loans. He converted a process of repossession into an art of towing away a car within forty-five seconds, a sort of legalized car theft. During these quick operations (they must be quick to avoid an altercation with an irate owner), he is focused, concentrated on his task, and extremely anxious. Approximately twenty to thirty minutes after the towing, he feels thirsty and extremely hungry. Mr. Zi has gained over thirty pounds in the span of two years, despite being reasonably active at work and in the gym. I believe that the anxiety of Mr. Zi's job caused his weight gain and that the treatment of anxiety and elimination of anxiety-provoking factors should come first, before any successful diet can be instituted.

**Question 3**. Every day I try to eat a light lunch, such as a salad or just a cup of soup. I feel fine for about an hour or two, but then I become terribly hungry. I can no longer concentrate on my work. I go through our large office searching for candies or cookies that many of my coworkers keep around. I tried bringing some fruit from home, but this didn't help; I was still extremely hungry. How shall I deal with my bouts of mid-afternoon hunger?

**Answer 3.** This is probably the biggest problem with dieting. Regardless of the type of diet we follow, when we become hungry it is very difficult to adhere to any program. Hunger is a dominant feeling. When we are really hungry, our mind is completely preoccupied with food. The thought of subsequent regret is driven away; the hunger prevails, and behavior is dominated by a search for food. We become overwhelmed by the hunger-driven inability to maintain our dietary program.

I must say at the outset, this problem is extremely common and there is nothing to be ashamed of. It is also a losing proposition trying to fight one's hunger by evoking the remnants of one's willpower. The only way to succeed is to change the environment in which we find ourselves at the time we feel hungry, to get away from food and to switch our mind to something completely different that can occupy us for a while.

I recommend that the minute you feel this uncontrollable hunger (after that small lunch that you were supposed to eat to stay on your diet) you leave your house, if you are at home. Go for a walk; go to the library, a bookstore, a department store, a museum—anywhere to be away from food and, better yet, where your mind can become engaged in a totally new activity, such as reading, analyzing, comparing, calculating, making plans, and so forth.

Certainly, this is much harder to do at work. When you remain hungry after lunch, sitting at your desk with your mind overwhelmed with thoughts of food, first try sipping water or a noncaloric drink. Frequently, small sips curb your feeling of hunger. If this doesn't help, a dozen almonds or a stick of string cheese is the next line of defense. Still the best approach to this residual hunger is to get truly busy and to be away from food.

Schedule a meeting, discuss work-related problems, get busy with manual tasks—do anything that takes your mind away from food.

**Question 4.** Someone told me that eating twice a day is the best way to lose weight. I tried this but found it difficult not to eat between breakfast and dinner. What is a good interval of time between meals?

**Answer 4.** I recommend that you eat every five to six hours during daytime. For example, eat at 800. AM, 1:00 PM, and 6:00–7:00 PM. I also stress that the time interval between the end of your dinner and your next breakfast be no less than twelve hours. If you finish your dinner at 8:00 PM, do not eat your breakfast before 8:00 the next morning.

**Question 5.** I've been looking for a diet that I can stick to without making a huge effort to find the "right" food items or perfect cooking style. What is the simplest and the most effective diet for a man who wants to lose ten to fifteen pounds?

**Answer 5.** The Draznin Calorie plan allows you to eat any grilled low-fat meat, poultry, or fish with most of the vegetables (except potatoes and corn) and a variety of fruit (except grapes and bananas). If you stay with these recommendations, you can lose ten to fifteen pounds within three months easily.

**Question 6.** I weigh 265 lb and I have type 2 diabetes that I am treating with a total of 114 units of insulin taken in three separate injections. I am ready to go on a strict low-calorie diet. How do I adjust my insulin? Do I stop it altogether?

**Answer 6.** Most likely you can cut your insulin dose in half without any problems, provided you are serious about trimming your food intake and you measure your blood sugar levels four times a day. Several years ago my colleagues and I conducted a study in which we recommended our overweight diabetic patients fast for five days, drinking only noncaloric fluids, before initiating dietary therapy. These patients did not take any insulin during this complete five-day fast, and they resumed taking it afterward depending upon their blood-sugar readings. These patients did very well, and only half of them required insulin after this initial fast. The danger arises if you reduce your insulin dose but do not reduce what you eat and do not check your blood-sugar levels. Clearly, working with your doctor or diabetes educator is preferable to doing it alone.

**Question 7.** I am five feet six inches and weigh 208 lb. I am taking two pills for my lipids, two for diabetes, two for high blood pressure, one aspirin, and multivitamins. I have recently gained seven pounds, and my blood sugar is just above 200 mg/dl. I was told to start taking another medication that might prevent absorption of sugars. Is there another way to achieve better control of my problems without so many pills?

**Answer 7.** Losing weight will help tremendously. Most likely your diabetes will improve, and quite likely your blood pressure and lipids will also improve. You seem to be a prime candidate for the Draznin Plan if you are ready to embark on this program. I also recommend meditation classes for mild hypertension and for learning to take control of your problems.

**Question 8.** I work out in the gym three times a week, and I cut down on the carbohydrates in my diet. I am really trying to eat healthy—fruits and vegetables. I drink a lot of fruit juices, not sodas—four to six glasses of orange or cranberry juice a day. Yet I have lost only two pounds in the last four months. Is there anything else I should be doing?

**Answer 8**. Unfortunately, yours is a common mistake. Fruit juices are extremely caloric, with simple sugars accounting for most of the calories. I firmly recommend that any fluid you consume (except for milk) should contain *no* calories. Stopping fruit juices would be my immediate recommendation.

**Question 9**. I followed your program for over six months, and I lost eighteen pounds. I now weigh 192 lb, down from 210. I walk an hour every day, but during the last three weeks I haven't lost any more weight. How do I get on the weight-losing track again?

**Answer 9**. An excellent question. Remember, the first goal of the Draznin Plan is to help you lose about 10% of your initial weight and maintain the reduced weight for about six to twelve months. At this point, one must reevaluate the program and make the next step. For example, if you are not doing three Draznin Miles a day, you should make an effort to get to this goal. If you do, you might want to increase your walking or jogging speed or possibly extend the time by an additional ten minutes a day. You can add 2,000 steps daily or be a little stricter about your diet.

**Question 10**. I have learned to take boredom out of my daily walks—I listen to books on tape as I stroll through our neighborhood, around a small park, and back home. It works well. It's the dietary part that I find more difficult to follow, simply because my choices are somewhat limited. In other words, the diet is boring. What would you suggest?

**Answer 10.** I would recommend expanding the variety of meat or fish you are buying and of the vegetables you eat. There are wonderful recipes in vegetarian cookbooks that you can adopt as well as numerous types of fish and nonfat meat that you can grill or sear. Adding various spices may also help.

**Question 11.** My blood-sugar levels hover around 220 mg/dl. My doctor tried me on three different medications, but they didn't seem to help. My weight is 190 lb, and my doctor tells me that unless I lose weight, he will have to start me on insulin. Is there anything else I can do?

**Answer 11.** Your doctor is absolutely correct to suggest that controlling your blood sugar is your number one priority. However, you can help yourself and your doctor to accomplish this task by losing weight. In this case, you may avoid insulin altogether. A lot of control over your health in your own hands.

**Question 12.** My twenty-two-year-old daughter weighs 186 lb and is only five feet four inches tall. Most importantly, however, she refuses to do anything about her weight. She says she feels good about herself, enjoys her friends and her lifestyle, and is proud to be who she is. On the one hand, I am glad she is not depressed and that she maintains her self-confidence; on the other hand, I am very much concerned and don't know how to help her. Your advice?

**Answer 12.** Unfortunately, your ability to help is limited at this point. A direct discussion or repeated confrontations will not help. You might work indirectly, so to speak. Invite her for walks, hikes, bike rides, or a swim. Change the way you cook at home, and, it is hoped, she will like the new recipes. Suggest that she consult a psychologist, perhaps for some other reason (if such exists), and then recommend to your daughter that she talk with the psychologist about her weight. This is not an easy task; it will certainly take some time, but being concerned about it is the first step.

**Question 13**. If I have a question about my weight maintenance or my diabetes, how can I contact you?

**Answer 13**. You can find me at the University of Colorado Health Sciences Center. In addition, you can obtain valuable information from numerous excellent Web sites related to diabetes, appropriately led by the American Diabetes Association (www.diabetes.org), the Juvenile Diabetes Federation (www.jdf.org), the International Diabetes Federation (www.idf.org), the British Diabetes Association (www.diabetes.org.uk), and the Joslin Diabetes Center (www.joslin.harvard.edu).

# Resources

**American Diabetes Association**
ATTN: National Call Center
1701 North Beauregard Street
Alexandria, VA 22311
1-800-DIABETES
www.diabetes.org

**American Dietetic Association**
120 South Riverside Plaza, Suite 2000
Chicago, IL 60606-6995
1-800-877-1600
www.eatright.org

**American Heart Association**
National Center
7272 Greenville Avenue
Dallas, TX 75231
1-800-AHA-USA-1
www.americanheart.org

**American Society for Nutrition**
9650 Rockville Pike
Bethesda, MD 20814
1-301-634-7050
www.nutrition.org

**Joslin Diabetes Center**
One Joslin Place
Boston, MA 02215
1-617-732-2400
www.joslin.org

**National Diabetes Information Clearinghouse**
1 Information Way
Bethesda, MD 20892-3560
1-800-860-8747
www.diabetes.niddk.nih.gov/

**NAASO, The Obesity Society**
8630 Fenton Street, Suite 918
Silver Spring, MD 20910
1-301-563-6526
www.naaso.org

# Index